THE

PEOPLE

IN

MY

HIPS

by

Ken Wolf

Introduction

The People in my Hips is my story.

It is a story that took me two years to tell because
I was so afraid that people would think that I was crazy.

I finally shared my story (with real video of my
experience) in my one man play THE PEOPLE IN MY
HIPS which was performed in NYC at Manhattan
Repertory Theatre, Jan. 17, 2009 through April 18, 2009.

Each night, as I recounted my crazy tale, presenting
real video of my "People in my Hips" experience that
I had self-filmed over three years, I would say to myself
"What the hell am I doing? What the hell am I doing?"

How in God's name could I share this?

But, you see, I had to...

When The People in my Hips first manifested, as I was
struggling to find a cure, I made a commitment to myself
that I would indeed cure myself and then help people
with similar problems by creating a movie or a play
and by going on The Oprah Winfrey Show. This crazy
commitment to help others was what kept me going,
kept me from taking drugs, kept me from despair. The
commitment that I made to tell this story to the world,
saved me.

Remarkably, I received rave reviews.

I'm a Personal Trainer, Yoga Instructor, Playwright and Actor.

I started Yoga Teacher Training in August 2002 at BeYoga (since sold to Yogaworks) in Westchester and New York City. For over a year, as I trained intensely in Yoga, my body started to remember things, things from my childhood I had since long forgotten, and physically, my body tried to help me remember.

And then, all hell broke loose!

I developed severe PTSD (Post Traumatic Stress Disorder) and I developed Multiple Personalites in my Hips.

I'm not kidding.

My body would cramp up unexpectedly, I would shake and cry, (especially during Yoga,) and, at other times, I could communicate with a child part of me from long ago (whom I dubbed "Baby Ken") who was living in my hips along with someone (or something else) who shall remain nameless at present.

I know this sounds crazy.

And it is.

But I am NOT crazy, and have never been crazy.

What I experienced was not mental illness. It was a physical/emotional energy imbalance that I was unable to control. Through my "insane" perseverance in my quest to heal, after three years I discovered a way to physically balance my imbalance, and inadvertently, through a bizarre sequence of events, I found a way to cure myself.

It is time we all look at "mental illness" differently.

Why I have to tell this story...

As I mentioned above, what kept me going during my three year process of trying to heal myself from the People in my Hips was the commitment that I made to myself that someday I would heal myself and then help others with this information. I am not a doctor. I am just a Personal Trainer, Yogi, Playwright and Actor. But what I discovered in my journey is profound.

I was a mess. My body was bouncing around by itself. My hips would cramp up repeatedly, I would be continually crying for what seemed like no reason, and a child part of me was taking over my body and telling me strange cryptic things. It really is unbelievable.

I moved out of the apartment that I was sharing with my girlfriend, and I moved to a little cottage up in the boondocks of northern Westchester. Part of me felt I was losing my mind, but part of me persevered - the still strong voice inside me, call it my soul, call it my inner voice, or call it God, but whatever you want to call it, this still strong voice inside me refused to believe in anything but possibility, that someday, somehow I would cure myself of my crazy condition and I would help others with this knowledge. My play THE PEOPLE IN MY HIPS was the first piece of this process. My PEEPS website and blog was the second piece and this book, now the third.

I was so scared to tell anyone about my condition. What was happening to my body was insane. I would be walking thru the Gym and all of a sudden I would be thrown into the wall by "The People in my Hips". An old, brutally beaten part of me was acting up and causing my life to turn upside down.

And now, thank God for it.

It is years later. I am so much better in so many ways.

Now that I have healed my condition, it is time to reach out and create a community where it is safe to share what other people might think crazy. These thoughts, these physical manifestations and feelings related to PTSD are just that - thoughts, bodily somatic responses and feelings.

They are not who we are.

They are not a label called CRAZY.

They are simply the process of our body/mind going about trying to heal itself.

Real Video of "the Peeps"

When I first manifested The People in my Hips, I started filming myself talking about my condition, and then I went on to film Yoga sessions where I shook and flew about the room. I even filmed psychotherapy sessions with my therapist "Dr. Freud" (Name changed so as to not freak out his clients.) In many of these sessions, I bounced, shook, and talked with "Baby Ken" in real time and cried, and cried, and cried. Filming my condition grounded me, kept me going, literally kept me alive, focused on a solution, even when the going got bad.

And it did get bad...

This real video of my experience can be found on at YOUTUBE channel: peopleinmyhips. There are a lot of videos there and it can be used as a supplement to this book. Please check it out. It is fascinating.

People are afraid to talk about this stuff. And I know for a fact that there are individuals out there who deal with this type of thing (maybe not as extreme) on a daily basis.

Old feelings manifesting in the present moment are not something to be frightened of.

They are something to EMBRACE.

Even sometimes, something to celebrate.

No more hiding.

It is time to talk openly, honestly and unafraid.

This book is dedicated to
the millions of sufferers of PTSD
and mental disease across the globe.
There are solutions.
There is another way to look at things.
Never give up.

CHAPTER ONE

My name is Ken Wolf. I am a playwright, an actor, the artistic director of Manhattan Repertory Theatre in New York City, and by day, a personal trainer and Yoga instructor. This is the story of my three year battle with The People in my Hips.

The story I am about to share with you is absolutely true. As a playwright, I write stories based on my life. I take crazy stories about my relationships, or crazy stories about my family and I put them up on stage, often just changing the names. Now I don't have many friends and my family hates me, but I do good work.

This story is very different. This story is a crazy story about about battling the crazy in me, about literally striking back at demons from a childhood which I never knew existed. It's about struggling in the MASH PIT of my mind for three long years as I embraced a past long forgotten.

When I was 10 years old, my father had a nervous breakdown and was admitted to ST. Vincent's Psychiatric Hospital in Harrison, NY where he received shock

therapy. I don't remember much about that time, but I do remember the ceramic ashtrays that he sent home from his arts and crafts class every couple of weeks.
And I didn't even smoke. For most of my adult life, I feared that someday I would "lose it" and go crazy and be put away like Dad. This story is a celebration of the fact that I will never ever live out my father's crazy legacy. Through my People in my Hips process, the story I am about to share with you, I have literally re-wired by body and my consciousness.

One of the things that kept me going during my crazy three year struggle with The People in my Hips, was the commitment I made to one day tell this story as a play or a movie. When The People in my Hips first manifested, I immediately started a video diary where I filmed myself talking about the "crazy" stuff happening in my life. Repeatedly, on these video diary entries, I made a commitment to Oprah to heal myself, and get on her show to help people with similar problems world wide. I also filmed psychotherapy, bodywork and Yoga sessions. Documenting my process with video was one of the ways I survived. Knowing that I would bear witness and someday tell this story, and hopefully help lots of people with similar problems was how I made it through. It's one of the reasons why I am writing this now in my right mind.

Three years ago, I healed myself of The People in my Hips. I had finally lived out and completed the story, and I had my theatre in which to present the story, yet I procrastinated on putting the show together because I was scared. I was scared that The People in my Hips might return, and scared that after sharing this material publicly, the world at large might think me mad, an extension of the craziness of my father. So I put off presenting the show telling myself I was too busy running my theatre to do tell this story.

And then one night, something happened which made me realize that I had to tell this story and tell it right away.

I was house managing for a Manhattan Rep play. While cleaning up in my office, I discovered a diary from 2005 that I had kept about The People in my Hips. I mostly did video diaries but this was about 30 pages of a written journal. This is what I read:

"I decided to relax my hip in therapy today, let it go and follow it to see what we could discover.

Immediately I started to bounce and shake and then my right hand started hitting my right leg repeatedly. Why was I hitting myself?

I went further into the memory. Something bad was happening. Something bad. I am being held down.

Who was it? Who was it?

It was Dark Man.

I can't tell anyone.

He said he would kill me if I told.

I HAD TO KEEP IT A SECRET - WAY DOWN IN MY HIPS!

I had to keep it a secret from EVERYONE.

Even myself… or I would die!

MY body is telling me the truth, showing me physically so that I will believe it…for I destroyed the memory years ago to survive.

WHAT BETTER WAY TO KEEP A SECRET? MAKE YOURSELF FORGET!"

I set the journal down.

I was stunned for I had absolutely no recollection of this event,

this therapy session

or of ever having written this journal.

And therein hangs a tale…

CHAPTER TWO

BeYoga Yoga Teacher training was a little challenging for my forty-four year old bones, but I stepped up to the plate and did remarkably well. The only problem that I experienced in my first couple of months of training was this strange lower back "burning." It wasn't a muscle pull or a spasm. It was like there was a lit cigarette trapped in muscles of my lower back right where my hip flexors connected to my lower spine. I attributed it to over training and I was fine with it.

But the truth of the matter is this...
I was pregnant with THE PEOPLE IN MY HIPS.

It was my third month of Yoga Teacher Training. I was taking a class at BeYoga in midtown Manhattan which was taught by an extremely gifted Yoga teacher by the name of Douglass Stewart. I had taken his class a number of times before and I loved it. His teaching style personified Yoga. He was present, compassionate and at times, humorous. Little did I know at this time, that we would form a unique YOGA BOND in the years to come.

It was towards the end of the class, and we were doing a Yoga Asana called Maltese Twist. It is a chest opener and a hip opener. One lies on their side, with their knees to their chest and then the upper torso twists open. As I moved into the twist, I started to cry... but I had no idea what I was crying about. Tears were streaming from my eyes, I was breathing as if I was crying, yet the crying was disconnected somehow. It was as if someone else was crying, while I stood by watching. It was bizarre. Unsettling.

As I moved out of the stretch, my "crying" subsided.

I talked with Douglass about it after class. He said that sometimes in the process of your Yoga practice feelings will arise. I should just breathe, relax and eventually the feelings will dissipate.

But that wasn't the case this time...

I was giving birth.

CHAPTER THREE

I didn't let my rather bizarre "crying experience" in class with Douglass keep me from my yoga teacher certification. I continued to train passionately in Yoga....

and, I continued to cry.

Now hold it a second.

Isn't Yoga supposed to calm you down?
Help you relax?

My experience with Yoga soon evolved into the exact opposite. It seemed like in every class I took, at some point in time, I would break into disconnected tears. My body would sob as I simply witnessed.

I soon began to notice a pattern. The biggest "cries" would occur when I was stretching my hip flexors. The hip flexors start on your upper leg and connect through your pelvis to your lower spine. It was almost as if my hip flexors were a direct line to my unconscious.

In the Yogic tradition, they say that there are seven Chakras or ENERGY WHEELS in the body. The seven chakras are aligned more or less along our spinal cord. When I first started to experience my disassociated sobbing, I researched the chakras to see if I could learn something that might help. My hips flexors literally passed thru the second chakra Svadisthana. This is what I discovered.

Svadisthana is related to our *sensing abilities, inner child issues and issues related to feelings.*

Now to be honest, I am not one of those people who believes everything that they read or are taught. During my Yoga training I questioned everything until I could experience validity or a reality to it. At this point in this story, I had been a personal trainer and fitness instructor for over 20 years. My "body" belief system was this: The body consists of muscles and bones, organs, blood and nerves.

CHAKRAS? CHAKRAS? If there are Chakras?

Show me one!

It was March, a Wednesday night. I was taking Yoga class taught again by Douglass Stewart. We were coming to the hip opening section of the class, and I SO DIDN'T WANT TO CRY but I decided that if I did begin to cry,

I wouldn't resist it. I would go into it, ask questions, try to learn more.

As I breathed into the hip opener, (ankle to knee asana) I started to shake a little, and then in a tidal wave of disassociated angst, the sobbing began. My head started to shake softly side to side as tears sprang from my eyes.

"What is all this about?" I asked my body. "Did someone do something to you? What happened? Did someone do something to you? Who did this?"

And then, (I tremble as I write this,) I **HEARD** a little voice from deep inside my body:

"It was Grampa. Grampa Wolf. He did it! He did it!"

I pulled out of the posture, stunned. I quickly lay down on my back on my mat, and quietly wept, hoping that no one in the class would see me.

"It was Grampa. Grampa Wolf. He did it! He did it!"

My Grandfather came to America from Germany in the 1940's. He lived with my Grandmother Katrina and his son Henry (my father), in Astoria Queens. To my knowledge, he worked as a waiter at the Glen Isle Casino and other places in the Metropolitan area. He was an alcoholic. He died of a stroke when I was 4 years old.

I have only one memory of him. He wore Dentures. He would take them out of his mouth and chase me and my older brother Mike around the house saying that he was going to bite us.

After my grandmother passed away in 1989, my four siblings and I went to her apartment in Astoria to go through her stuff, take the things that we wanted and give away the rest. I took nothing, except for …

Grampa's dentures.

Gramma had kept them for over 26 years.

Why I took them, I have no idea.

"Grampa, what did you do?

What the fuck did you do?"

CHAPTER FOUR

I was considerably shaken by the "child voice" I heard in Yoga class that day. It was bizarre. Something was wrong. I needed to know what was going on in me. And what the hell happened in my past? Did my Grandfather do something to me? Or was that "child voice" just a figment of an overly emotional imagination?

I talked with Douglass after the class and made arrangements to train with him privately to get to the bottom of this mystery inside of me. The next day, Douglass and I met at my apartment on the Upper West Side of Manhattan.

When Douglass arrived, we sat cross-legged on our Yoga mats in my living room and I told him my tale of disassociated woe. There was something so peaceful and safe about his demeanor. He listened compassionately until I was all talked out, and then, we began our YOGA.

We started with an Arching Cat asana and I immediately started to cry, again totally disassociated from any connection with the emotion. Douglass quietly watched. I pushed up into Downward Dog but the shaking was too much so Douglass gently rolled me on my side for a supported Maltese Twist, and that is when I started... to remember! Maybe it was Douglass's gentle touch or the safety of being in my home, but for the first time my sobbing emotions were connected - AND THEY WERE CONNECTED TO EVERYTHING!

I was five, I felt/saw my Father kicking me as I lay on the kitchen floor - I was four, almost drowning in the Long Island Sound at Playland in 1962 - I was thirteen being beat up by Roger Fenton in Mill Pond Park - I was one, someone was holding me by the neck as an infant and smashing my head into the floor again and again and again! And as Douglass gently moved me into various supported Yoga stretches, a universe of memories unfolded like a motion picture manifesting through my body, shaking me, moving me. Some images/feelings were from my conscious memory, other images/feelings were brand new as if they didn't belong to me or to my past.

And as I stretched with the gentle assist of Douglas, I could feel the utter fear of waiting to be belted in the bathroom by my father, the sad melancholy of having to go into 6th grade knowing that my parent's were divorced making me a subhuman child, and the paralyzing new memory at four years of age, hiding from my rageful father in a closet in a garment bag fearing that he would kill my mother, my brothers and sisters and then me.

And I cried, and I shook and I shook and I cried and with Douglass's gentle assist I did Yoga....Yoga unlike any Yoga I had ever experienced before!

WHAT THE HELL WAS GOING ON?

We eventually stopped. I lay there a blathering amoeba of emotion splattered on my living room floor.

And Douglass sat quietly watching.

It had been so real... yet so unreal.

And as I lie there as human emotional protoplasm, I knew that the worst was yet to come...

CHAPTER
FIVE

Douglass and I met again the following week.
I had been to Yoga class four times in between our last
session, and in each class, emotion arose in my body/
consciousness but not as intensely as in the privacy of my
apartment. I was scared out of my mind as to what might
manifest that day.

We began our Yoga and the emotional roller coaster
resumed again. I immediately started to shake as we
began with simple Sun Breaths. Douglass then took me
down on to the floor for various assisted Yoga stretches
and I immediately started to cry and almost
hyperventilate still not knowing what it was all connected
to.

And then, the BODY MOVIE began again, like a flip
book of hundreds of emotional moments from, not just
my childhood, but from my entire life.

Breaking up with my girlfriend Janet in 8th grade, fist
fighting with my brother Mike at ten years of age, being
pulled from underneath my bed and then being beaten by

my father at age eight, falling down and spraining my knee at eighteen and on and on and on.

I was fascinated and scared, amazed and so confused.

Somehow through Yoga I had opened a Pandora's box of emotion somehow being released through my body. I shook and cried, hyperventilated and wailed.

And this was YOGA?
Isn't Yoga supposed to calm you down?

And then, I **WAS** my father, pleading with my mother seeking-needing her approval, and then I **WAS** my sister Cathy - something had happened to her, I/she was so sad, so so sad. Then I was hiding with her, at maybe seven years of age. My parents were fighting in the kitchen, yelling, screaming - we had to protect ourselves!

Keep the door closed! Keep the door closed!

Again, it was all so vivid and confusing, scary, violent and sad. An emotional collage of terror, love lost and physical violence. What the hell was happening? Why was I being shown all this? Yes, some of it was from my conscious memory but some memories were mysteries unfolding before me, so new, so alive and so so frightening!

I **WAS** my mother terrified running my five children into the Rambler station wagon to escape from the crazy man - my father. And I was me at eight years of age, with a 102 fever in the back seat, crying, screaming for my life.

"Where are we going? Where are we going?"

Meanwhile, I am bouncing, shaking, wailing on my living room floor. I wasn't doing it. Something was doing it to me. The old memories, they were here now happening in my body, in my mind, somehow alive again!

"Please stop! Please stop oh GOD PLEASE STOP!!!"

....

Douglass is gently pulling on my legs and moving them gently side to side, releasing my hips. Our session is ending.

As I lay there, dizzy from the flash flood of emotion in my body, I can feel something...
a thought,
a presence in my left hip,
a tightness, a piece of...
a piece of...

fear...

somehow wanting, needing to be heard,

needing to be expressed,

to be set free...

...***trapped*** in my left hip.

"Oh God, please help me. Please help me."

Douglass left. I needed some caffeine. Boy, did I need caffeine, and even more so...

I needed CAKE! Chocolate cake if possible.

As I was walking down the block, on my way to Starbucks to feed my craving, I ran into my girlfriend, Jen who lived with me, who was coming home from work.

"How'd it go with Douglass?" she said with a smile.

"It was unbelievable." I replied as I felt a cold tremor in my left hip.

Yes, it was fear.

CHAPTER SIX

"Ahhhhhhhhh!!"

I awoke with a start. My right hip flexor was locked up. I was in agonizing pain.

It was 2 weeks after I started my one on one Yoga work with Douglass.

"Ahhhhhhhhh!!" again I moaned as I tried to move.

"What is it? Are you Ok?" my girlfriend stammered also waking from a deep sleep.

"Yeah,…I'm fine. It's just a cramp. I will be fine."

I crawled out of our bed and crawled on the floor out of the bedroom into the living room.

"You're not Ok!" she called after me.

"Yeah, I'm fine. It is just a cramp." I whispered back from the living room floor as I lay on my back pulling my right knee to my chest. Tears were falling from my eyes. My head was shaking side to side. There was no connection to the emotion. It was my **STUFF** attacking me in my sleep. Why was it doing this? What the hell was going on?

It was 3:30 a.m. I was due to get up at 5 a.m. for I had a 6 a.m. client in Westchester. How the hell was I going to work this cramp out and get to work on time? I pulled both my knees into my chest and rolled my bent legs in my hips sockets.

"AHHHHHHHHH SHIT!"

My lower back cramped again.

My head now was rocking back and forth by itself as if my body was saying "**NO**!"

I was hyperventilating, and again, the tears were falling. I crawled into the bathroom, still in great pain, my body shaking. I turned on the tub.

"Are you OK?" from the bedroom.

"Yes, I'm fine. I'm fine. It is just a cramp. I will be fine."

I crawled into the bathtub, and then, laying on my side in six inches of hot water, I bent my knees and reached back and grabbed my ankles (like doing the Yoga Bow Asana only on my side) and I lay there crying, the shaking from my head almost splashing the water out of the tub.

I stayed in the tub for almost an hour, rolling and shaking. It started to release.

I pulled myself out, managed to dry myself off, and them back in my underwear, I crawled back out to the living room where I continued to stretch. I needed to be out of there in less than thirty minutes.

My girlfriend Jen, probably hearing the sound of my head shaking side to side on the floor, got out of bed and joined me in the living room.

"Are you OK?"

"Yeah, just a cramp. Ummm, could you just put your foot on my pelvis here?

"What?'

"Can you just help me stretch this out? Just put your foot on the left side of my pelvis here."

"Are you Ok?"

"Yeah, just put your foot here." I said pointing toward the top left part of my pelvis.

She placed her foot on the left top part of my pelvis as I held my right knee to my chest.

"Now push down, hard. Step on me."

"Are you Ok?" I could see the love and great concern in her eyes.

"Yes, I'm fine. This will help. Please."

She pressed down with her foot. I held my neck tightly so that it wouldn't shake. My head quivered slightly.
I could feel a burning sensation through my lower back.

"Are you Ok?"

"Yeah, Yeah, that's good, that really helps. Now can you do the other side?"

Needless to say, I was able to get to work and function, still in some pain, but I hid it well.

But I didn't hide it well enough from Jen.

She was scared.

CHAPTER SEVEN

I am cramped up. I can barely walk. Douglass just arrived at my apartment for our Yoga session. He is rolling out the mats on the living room floor.

"I don't know how much I can do. I cramped up today after Spin class - my hip flexor is locked again. Douglass, this sucks." I sighed seeking his sympathy.

"So let's do something different." He said with a wink. "I think we have done enough bouncing lately."

"Absolutely! So what do you want to do?" I was nervous.

"Why don't we sit and breathe and I will take you on a guided meditation through your Chakras?"

"Sure. Why not." I replied smiling, but I was so damn scared. Whenever Douglass and I worked together, my practice became a direct live wire to my unconscious and... **Fireworks!**

Little did I know at the time, that that session would be a **_NUCLEAR EXPLOSION!_**

We sat cross-legged on our mats facing each other. Arms out, back of our wrists to our knees, palms open, my thumbs and my first fingers were touching in Jnana Mudrā.

Douglass began his guided meditation starting with the base chakra MULADHARA, bringing my awareness to the area down below the base of my spine.

My breath shortened.

"Breathe, Ken, breathe."

I suddenly felt dizzy. Douglass continue inviting me to bring my awareness/explore my experience of this area. I started to hyperventilate. Douglass asked me to bring white light into this area, peace, calm, healing white light. My breath shortened even more. My body started to slightly hop up and forward while I sat there cross-legged. Douglass then invited me to bring that white light into my second Chakra **SVADISTHANA**, and I immediately started to involuntarily shake forward and back.

"Are you alright, Ken?"

"Yes, Yes, I'm fine. Let's go. Keep going."

My body started to shake harder forward and back, back and forth, I could feel pain, sharp pain at the very base of my spine by my genitals.

"Oh Fuck!"

"Ken?"

"Keep going Douglass, I am fine."

I started to bounce harder and harder. Suddenly, I could see Resurrection Church where I was an altar boy, or was I, was that just the Kindergarten pageant where I was the altar boy? Why is that priest telling me to come and serve mass? Fuck this is like a bad Access Hollywood segment? A Priest? That's been done! What the hell is really real here?

Douglass then led me to the third Chakra MANIPURA, stomach, fire, energy center, and then there came a cry… a cry, a howl… a howl from the darkest depth of hell, a child's cry, a child at the age of six or seven howling, *HOWLING* for his life, Oh God, not again! No more please no more!

"Ken, are you alright?"

"Yes, keep going."

I need to know, I need to know. I need to know. I need to know.

And so Douglass led me through the remaining Chakras:

ANAHATTA, the Heart Chakra.

NO DON'T PLEASE STOP! PAIN. PAIN. PAIN.
Don't leave me!
Don't stay!
Go away! Let me go away!

"Keep going, Douglass."

VISHUDDHA, the Throat Chakra.

SUDDENLY I was drowning.

I can't breathe. I can taste the salt water in me, in my lungs, I was gasping I am gasping for my life. I heard/hear a cry. It was me, Younger, lost, crying, Am I going to die? Help me. Help me.
"Ken?"
"Keep going Douglass!"

AJNA, the Third Eye Chakra.

Centered above my brow. Intuition. All was black. I am panting. In the dark. I am in the closet.

NO, don't do it. No, please! No, don't!

SAHASRARA, the Crown Chakra -

WHERE IS THE WHITE LIGHT? WHERE IS THE FUCKING WHITE LIGHT? THE GOD DAMNED HEALING LIGHT! WHERE?

My body is bouncing forward and back. My head is shaking 100 miles a second back and forth like the Energizer Bunny on speed, and I am hyperventilating.

Tears, buckets, oceans of wet pain, fly and fall across the room. I am seeing things and I don't know what I am seeing and I know they are bad. No, not bad! Evil!

And then, I'm crying, wailing, howling, howling from the darkest depths, from the Forgotten Land deep inside,

HELPME HELPME HELPME HELPME!!!

...oh my ...God.

The hair is standing on the back of my neck.
My breathing slows. I am quietly weeping. Douglass sits across from me watching, calm and curious.

This is nuts. This is nuts. This is nuts.

Our guided meditation...
It felt and looked as if I was being raped.

CHAPTER EIGHT

My second 200 hour round of Yoga Teacher Training went on hiatus for the Summer. We still had to get in our quota of classes but I didn't have to attend any seminars or workshops with the group until September.

Thank God.

There was something wrong in me.

I needed to figure this one out.

The last couple of weeks I had been distracted at our Yoga meetings, uncomfortable. I wasn't ready to share what was happening to me with the group. I was the only man in our training. And probably the only Yogi with People in his Hips.

My hips continued to lock up almost every night, sometimes worse than other nights. I told Jen that it was probably the new mattress that we had been sleeping on since we moved in together. I said it was too soft. Part of me knew that the mattress wasn't the culprit, but part of me hoped and prayed that it was.

Please let it be the mattress!
Please let it be the mattress!
Please let it be the mattress!

I went out and got a bed - sized piece of plywood and placed it under our mattress.

AHHHHHHHHHHHH!

I awoke that night my hips in a spasm.

We placed a mattress pad over the mattress that would make it firmer.

AHHHHHHHHHHHH!

I awoke folded up like a pretzel in pain.

It wasn't the mattress. It was in me.
But how could I share this with my girlfriend?

"I'm sorry, there is stuff in me that makes it virtually impossible for me to sleep next to you."
Wow, that's one way to nurture a relationship.

Yet pretending that this hip issue wasn't an issue wouldn't nurture a relationship either.

But I pretended anyway…how could I explain this?
I am channeling in all known and unknown abusive events in my life during Yoga, and then, at night, when I dream, this stuff is somehow getting into my muscles and crippling me.

Also, I am starting to feel paranoid especially when a *MAN* is standing behind me on line, or sitting behind me on a train, and I am feeling very uncomfortable in general around older men.

Damn, this does not look good. What is going on? What the hell have I forgotten?

What happened to me as a child?

What secret horrific events are still somehow trapped in my body?

And how can I share all this with the woman I love? Could she ever understand if I don't even understand it?

So I dived into denial and it became all about the mattress. I became obsessionally obsessive about the board, the pad, the position I slept, and on and on, so needless to say, going to bed with my amazing girlfriend, soon became no fun. Plus the thought of "getting involved" with her and then having my head start shaking side to side like a jackhammer was so unsexy.

God bless her. She is such an amazing woman.
She tried so hard to understand and solve this "Mattress"

problem, but when I looked into her eyes, all I could see was the fear underneath. She knew something was wrong. Terribly wrong.

And I was too frightened to share the truth…

…the truth that I was coming undone.

CHAPTER NINE

The days that followed are some of the oddest days of my life. Normally, when one experiences emotion, there is a thought, or an image, or someone says something that triggers an emotional response. For me, I simply felt emotions now emulating from my hips, almost as if my hips were another person, or if they were talking to me, or if they weren't even connected to my body. I felt random emotions manifesting out of what seemed like nothing all. Random, totally messed up emotions channeling out of my hips.

As I taught class, I could feel "sad melancholy" emulating from my hips. As I drove home, I could feel the "tears of a sad little lost boy." Sometimes my hips would actually burn in the front, right and left as if someone was tearing their fingernails into my pelvis. And my hip crease, where the pelvis connects with the upper leg was almost always in a spasm. When I went to release it, stretch it, I would cry, shake and bounce.

I was so scared.

Meanwhile, my home life was falling apart. There was this unknown energy or entity somehow trapped between Jen and I which I had named "THE MATTRESS," or "MY TIGHT HIP." I couldn't talk about the emotional aspect, it made no sense, and if I went there, to Jen, it would looked like I was going mad.

In my soul, I knew I wasn't going nuts. There was no doubt. I knew it wasn't my mind. But there was some crazy energy/entity/memory in me demanding to be released and my BODY couldn't hold it in.

Was this a nervous breakdown?
Was I recreating my father's legacy?
Was it time for my shock therapy?

For most of my adult life, I feared that someday, I too would lose it, go crazy like Dad and be sent away. Was this that moment? My self-fulfilling prophecy manifesting out of YOGA catapulting me into the fucked up footsteps of my crazy father?

Before we go any further, I just want to give you a little backstory about my father so you can better understand this tale. My memories of Dad are two-fold and that was the problem. When I was young, he was a tyrant, angry and unavailable. After St. Vincent's and his shock therapy, he and my mother divorced, and something happened in him. He saw the abusive person that he had become, and he vowed to change and to dedicate himself to truly loving his five children to make amends for his abusive behavior. He went back to the Church. He studied scripture, and he did everything in his power to bring joy into our lives. We became his raison d'etre, his reason to live.

And he became the father, I always dreamed of.

He died in 1989 of a heart attack.

Yes, I remembered and understood that he beat me when I was young.
But was there more?

NO! NO! NO! NO!
I LOVE YOU, DADDY!

So now there was this mystery in me. Somewhere, sometime in my past, really crazy things happened to me. I had no real conscious memories of these events, but my hips were somehow trying to communicate with me.

My hips were trying to communicate with me?

Yes, or the emotion in the hips, or the energy trapped in my hips, or the entity in my hips, whatever you would like to call it.

THAT'S NUTS!

A whole new past was unfolding before me. What the hell happened to me as a child? Was I really raped? And what the heck was happening in my body?

And deep down inside, I knew what was coming out of my hips was real. Coming out, maybe not in a proper order, or the proper cognitive packaging, but it was coming out. And it was real - the CREEPY MONSTERS and The DARK MEN that I made myself FORGET in order to survive...

oh please, no...

CHAPTER TEN

As I was *"coming undone."* I got really good at pretending that everything was Ok. Some days while teaching my core class when I was in the "hip cramp" mode, I would simply not demonstrate, because if I demonstrated on the floor I knew I would not be able to get back up to standing, or I would start to channel in bizarro feelings which would not be good for my fitness business. With Jen, I would simply say my hip was tight and reference something inane about getting a new mattress.

There is this strange thing about **NOT TELLING THE TRUTH,** (which isn't necessarily lying, but just as bad.) **NOT TELLING THE TRUTH** creates walls. First the walls are small and transparent, but as one continues to **NOT TELL THE TRUTH** the walls soon become big and solid and unbreakable. **NOT TELLING THE TRUTH** does not foster intimacy in any way. It fosters *PRETEND. DENIAL.* Ultimately, it fosters *EMPTINESS.* **NOT TELLING THE TRUTH** is lonely, selfish, but sometimes temporarily *SAFE.*

I told myself I needed that safety to figure things out. To fix myself. To somehow make things better before it all fell apart…   WHAT THE HELL WAS I THINKING?

My condition, whatever it was, whatever was coming out of me was ultimately a manifestation of my body **NOT TELLING THE TRUTH** of what really happened to me as a child. As I trained in Yoga, I inadvertently opened a floodgate of truth, which was so outside of my belief system as to what I thought was true. It made no sense. It was crazy. I needed to push it away. Keep it away.

This is not me. This is not who I am. This is not true. This in not really happening. It is the mattress. My relationship. My hip. My Yoga training.

I AM NOT RESPONSIBLE. I AM A VICTIM!

A victim. Maybe. Maybe in ways I could only imagine in my worst nightmares.

Whatever this energy was I would not let it WIN! I would fight back, fight back, fight back!

Can you see the really scary global metaphor here?

So I started "going to the mat" doing Yoga as often as I could to work this stuff out, which ultimately helped _bring_ it out. The feelings emanating from my hips became stronger. Sometimes I would just get nauseous. Other times, I would feel anxious and then fight with my girlfriend placing, assigning the feelings to her:

SHE IS DOING THIS TO ME!

Other times, I would pull back, eat pizza, cake, stuff it all down, get quiet, not talk, wander through bookstores aimlessly, often avoiding coming home until as late as possible and sometimes making up lame excuses and just staying up in my cabin in Westchester and not even coming home to New York City to sleep with the love of my life. Everything was wrong. I was scared, determined, lost and relentless. I knew and I didn't know.

Oh God, please help me!

No, I can do it. I can handle it alone.
I will not be beaten up again.

Oh please help me, Dad, Mom, Bro Mike, God, Food, Bookstores, Denial! Please anyone, anything please....

But no, ….not you…

no,

no,

no,

not you!

CHAPTER ELEVEN

It was September now.

My girlfriend Jen and I broke up. We had a couple conversations where I expressed we were just not right for each other **(NOT TELLING THE TRUTH)** and that we would be happier uncoupled **(NOT TELLING THE TRUTH!)**

I moved out. I moved full-time into my cottage in Northern Westchester, and life went on.

I was alone up in the woods, alone in my cabin,
safe,
        ....and scared.

Like a festering boil, it was all coming to a head...
        ...and there was nothing I could do to stop it.

My older sister Cathy is a psychologist so I called her and left a message saying I was having some emotional issues asking her to refer me to a good therapist. I also called ALEXANDER HAND, the head guru at BeYoga, who led some of my Teacher Training classes and I set up a private session with him.

My meeting with Alexander was at the 56th St studio where he had a private office. I entered, talked with the young girl at the desk and she sent me into his office. I rolled out my Yoga mat and sat cross-legged waiting for Alexander. A moment later, he entered. Alexander was short, a little over weight, with a long white beard and a charismatic smile.

"Namaste! How may I help you? he said with a wink.

I was freaking out. Would he even understand?

"Well, I have been having some problems in my hips."

Alexander jumped right in almost frightening me.

"Second Chakra Svadisthana: the Lesson - the RIGHT TO FEEL. Having emotional problems?"

"Yeah, sort of?"

"Well, sit, close your eyes and breathe."

I closed my eyes and took a deep breath.

"What do you feel?" Alexander whispered.

My head suddenly shakes side to side.

"Oh see that, you are blocked. AT YOUR HEART CHAKRA - ANAHATA. THE LESSON - the RIGHT TO LOVE. You need to forgive someone." He seemed very proud of himself with that response. Sounded like New Age gobblety-gook to me.

"Uh huh?" I responded.

"You are experiencing the classic PITA imbalance. Yoga prescription: Slow, silent practice every day, and each night before you go to bed, rub coconut oil over your entire body."

"What?"

"RUB COCONUT Oil over your entire body before you go to bed. It will help balance your pita. That and the forgiveness. Now let's do some MOOBEE Points on your back to help balance your energy."

"What are MOOBEE points?

"Energy points that I discovered intuitively. I never studied MOOBEE, I just knew. They should help balance your imbalance, that and the coconut oil "

I took off my shirt and lay on a small portable massage table in the room. Alexander then proceeded to press on certain points on my back, ...then as he was pressing on those points, the room started to spin.

OH NO NOT AGAIN PLEASE NO!!!!

I was again somehow transported back in time. It was dark, so so dark. I was being held down. I was scared so scared, someone, the dark man was holding me down. He was hurting me. My right leg started to kick violently. I tried to hold in a tortured scream but I couldn't. My entire body began to shake as Alexander continued to press on my back and neck.

OH HELL!

I wanted to yell out: *Please stop! Please stop stop!*
but part of me was hoping that whatever he was doing on
my back would heal me.

The past was *NOW NOW NOW NOW! HELP!*
and I was somehow trapped in it! *HELP!* fighting for
my life.......

    NOOOOOOOOOOOOOOOOOOO!!!!!

"There you go." Alexander murmured when we
finished and the energy finally dissipated. "That will be
$175 dollars. Please make your check out to cash."

My body lay on the massage table, trembling.

"And don't forget the COCONUT OIL."

CHAPTER TWELVE

That night, I put on a pair of old underwear, and broke out the coconut oil, which I had bought at a health food store that afternoon. I was actually going to cover my body with it in some insane hope that it would magically cure me. I broke out the video camera, flipped it on, and started my coconut bath.

I felt really dumb. I made jokes into the camera. I cried for a little bit, but basically, it was useless. (You can see the video on YOUTUBE channel : PeopleinmyHips. It is actually funny and sad at the same time.) After my greasy adventure, I took a long, hot bath and went to bed. I slept a fitful sleep.

The next day, I awoke early and there was this weird, wild energy flowing up and down my body, most of it centering around my pelvis. It felt like I had an electric lamp up my you know what. Something was wrong, very wrong.

It was getting worse.

"Oh my God, and I have to teach class today!"

I arrived early at the Community Center where I teach my classes. I was a mess. Energy and old feelings were flowing through my body and they were out of control. The director of the center was coming in. I pulled him aside.

"Jim, can I talk to you. You have a sec."

"Sure."

We went into his office. The tears streamed from my eyes like a mini-waterfall.

"Something is happening to me. I don't know what it is. I think I will be OK but I just want to give you a heads up in case I need your help.

"Are you alright, Ken?"

"Yeah, I am fine. It is just old stuff. Old stuff. I will be fine. But I just want to you to know that I am a little out of sorts in case I need your help."

"Are you sure you are going to be alright?"

"Yeah."

"Well, I am here if you need me. We all are here if you need anything."

"I'll be fine. I just wanted you to know…"

I was really scared, unnerved, distracted in class, unfocused, but I did my best to stay grounded.

"Focus on teaching, Ken. Focus on how you can help your students exercise better. Don't focus on you. Focus on teaching."

It was so weird. I could feel a tightness in my neck, squeezing and then it was gone. At times, it felt like the top half of my body was teaching class, while my lower body was weeping. A bizarre battle between my head and my emotions.

And my neck was so tight....

At the end of the class, as we were stretching, my head suddenly twitched side to side. I stopped it. No one noticed or said anything.

"Oh please not here!"

I was feeling so sad, almost sickly sad as I stretched and smiled and pretended.

"What the hell is going on? Please not now, not here..."

After class, I had two private clients.

"Oy, how am I going to do this?"

I pretended. I smiled. I motivated. I held it in.

"Oh please no not now! Do you hear me? NOT NOW PLEASE!!

On my way home that afternoon, I knew I had to do something. This was crazy. The feelings emanating from my hips were getting stronger and stronger. Something was coming out. Something bad. Someone or something was trying to communicate with me… or hurt me.

I knew who it was…but I didn't.

"Something is happening. I'm coming apart!"

There was some/one/thing in my hips, trying to talk to me, tell me things... or maybe just hurt me.

I had to do something. I had to make this better.

It was time.

Time to have a one-on-one conversation...

...with my left hip.

What the hell was I thinking?

CHAPTER THIRTEEN

I turned the camera on. I sat in my big easy chair.

"I don't know if this is going to work, if I am going to be able to connect with this part of me, but I have a feeling I will be able to." I said to the camera.

I then closed my eyes. I could feel the energy in my left hip emanating down to my left foot. I started to breathe slowly, softly, not Yoga breathing, normal people breathing. I had to relax, connect to this part of me, make it go away, oh please, make it go away. My head started to shake ever so slightly side to side as I tried to relax my body. My left foot started shaking violently and then it stopped, returning to a tiny tremor. I continued to try to relax. It was time to communicate, to talk to this part of me which was somehow emerging out of my body.

"Tell me who you are? What you are?" I thought to myself.

My legs started to shake again and then more, and more, and then I could feel the muscles of my jaw tighten and my head looked up and a sound, a cry emerged, from my throat, high-pitched and ...so so scared, like a child, a child version of myself, a baby version, a baby Ken whining crying sound emerged!

What happened back then?" I thought to myself, and my body immediately started to jump and rock as my legs shook.

"AHHHM, soooooo SCARED!!!" wailed out of me but not really out of me, out of my past, somewhere deep inside me. It's voice was high-pitched and frightening.

"Why are you so scared?" I thought and the Baby Ken part of me immediately responded with a frightening wail. The shaking got faster.

And then, my body started to bounce. Almost jump. I opened my eyes hoping that it would stop, but it didn't.

I started talking to the camera.

"Look at this! I am not doing this. It is doing it by itself. This is wild!"

My body started to literally jump up and down and my head went side to side as if it was being punched. The shaking got more violent as I bounced higher and more violently.

"I think I have stop, I have to ground, oh shit, I think I have to stop, ground."

I bring my hands into the yogic prayer position and breathe heavily. My body is no longer jumping but my legs are vibrating like I have five hundred volts of electricity surging through my body.

"I have to ground, ground, I have stop."

Slowly, I compose myself.. my body stills...

I am scared out of my mind.

My body started bouncing around violently by itself, with my eyes open, as I talked to the camera and communicated with some bizarre "Baby Ken" living in my hips! This was beyond me, utterly crazy!

And what could I do? Who could I tell about this? My legs and my body were bouncing around and I wasn't even doing YOGA! To be totally honest, despite my curious nature, I don't think I have ever been more scared in my life.

This was MENTAL INSTITUTION stuff. There was two of me, living in me. This was nuts, wrong, evil, sick, mental and so so scary! Something needed to be done.

So what did I do?

I continued to delve, explore, and go where I really shouldn't have been going. This whole experience was so outside of my belief system as to what was possible. How was my body moving of it's own accord? What the hell was splitting off in me? And the most frightening piece, WHAT HAPPENED TO ME as a young child which I have forgotten, and why is my body choosing this time (at age 45) to tell me the truth?

This was something out of a bad Sci-Fi flick.

The brutally beaten child-self is taking over the Personal Trainer's body to seek out and murder his abuser, dragging said Personal Trainer along for the ride.

(You will see as this story unfolds, there just might be some truth to this...)

Oh my God, help me...

CHAPTER
FOURTEEN

So my body started jumping around by itself as I communicated with a displaced "child-self" that was manifesting from my hips.

What the HELL?

My nervous system was on edge. My mind confused. There was some unknown event or events deep within me causing this "child-self" to try and communicate with me, and that communication stemming from my hips was causing me to come undone. Totally undone. I was losing it and I was so so so scared.

THIS IS CRAZY! THIS IS CRAZY STUFF!
Soon I will be making ashtrays like old Daddy-O!

My impulse was to do YOGA, ground with YOGA, maybe possibly, if I could connect so intensely intimately with my body, I could release or let go of this "craziness" that was manifesting in me and through me.

I made a commitment that I would not under any circumstances let myself BE COMMITTED. I would figure this out.

Fix it.
　　　Cure it.
　　　　　Break it!
　　　　　　　Whatever I had to do I would do it.

Deep inside, I was so clear that this experience or process or whatever this was would not be my one way ticket to the LOONEY BIN.

I WOULD NOT UNDER ANY CIRCUMSTANCES LIVE OUT MY FATHER'S LEGACY.

Thank God for clarity.

This clarity, this unfettered determination is what kept me going. The stubborn Capricorn goat in me would not let these feelings or this child self, or this experience win.

So I decided I needed to do EVERYTHING in my power to fix myself, to release this crazy energy and get back to a normal life.

I barely slept that night. I could feel the energy running up and through my abdomen. It was like the energy had a life of it's own.

I had to move some spin bikes for my classes that day so I rented a truck. As I was driving to pick them up, my teeth started to chatter and my head started to shake side to side. There was something about the movement of the truck which was bringing stuff up. Suddenly, and this is the God's honest truth, I felt two hands strangling me on the neck. But I was alone in the truck. And then I felt as if someone was punching me on the back. It was crazy. It was like I was split in two. Half of me was in the present moment driving a truck and the other half was in the 1960's being brutally attacked.

It was the DARK MAN, time traveling, coming back for more fun.....

Somehow I made it thru my day. Try moving 16 spin bikes in the rain while being strangled and beaten by invisible hands. Not fun!

And no one was there. It was all made up in my mind or coming out of my body, out of my hips, out of the crazy energy that I had somehow brought to life in my body. Sometimes the room would start to spin. It was almost as if I was being TIME TRAVELED back to another time AND I was here, present in this time, here with ANGRY HANDS choking me and ANGRY FISTS hitting me and ANGRY shoes kicking me in the back!

I called my sister again. I needed a therapist.
No answer again. I left another message.

DAMN! I need help! Something. Anything.

I couldn't wait. A number of years earlier when I was having some relationship issues, I had seen a psychologist named Susan Danvers. I found her number, called and left a message saying that I would drop off a DVD of my conversation with my displaced child self from the night before.

I dropped a DVD off that afternoon at her office and her receptionist called me and I made an appointment to see Susan that night.

I entered. Susan looked older, tired. She also looked scared.

I was a mess. I was shaking slightly and half-weeping as I entered. When last I saw Susan I was complaining about my girlfriend problems. This time, I had a displaced child self living in my hips and imaginary hands, choking me and hitting me. My how I have grown!

"Hi Ken, it's good to see you again. I got your call and your DVD." She smiled but I could see the fear.

"Did you watch it?" I asked.

"No, I didn't. I don't think I need to watch it."

She watched it. I could tell.

"It is only 5 minutes. Do you have a computer here?" I needed to know that she saw it. So she could see how messed up I am so she could somehow help me with all of her girlfriend problem advice!

"No, I don't think I need to watch it." Susan reiterated.

"Why?" I demanded. "It is what is going on for me! Maybe you could understand. Maybe you could help if you saw it!

"I don't need to see it."

Why was she being so confrontational? I need help! I need help!

"Why? Why don't you need to see it? If you haven't seen it, how do you know that you don't need to see it?"

"Seeing it is not going to help your therapy here." She said smugly.

"Why?" My head started to shake slightly up and down. My left hip started to burn. I could feel again the hands on my neck choking me choking me choking me.

"Everything happens in this room." She said calmly. "I don't need to see the DVD. It all happens in this room. So what is going on for you?"

I flipped!

"What is going on for me? I am pissed off that you won't take four minutes and look at my MENTAL BREAKDOWN on DVD. If you saw what was going on with me, maybe you could help me!!!!!!"

"I'm fine." She murmured calmly.

"What the fuck do you mean you are fine? What about me? I am the patient and I am not fine. I AM NOT FINE!"

"Ken, please calm down." She said assertively. "Obviously, you're upset."

"Uh yeah, wouldn't you be upset if all day long the invisible man was choking you and hitting you on the back?"

She sat there frozen and then whispered. "No one is choking you. You seem like you're fine."

"What?"

"You seem like you're fine."

Whatever was left in me of any semblance of rationality just flew out the window!

"I AM NOT FINE!" I screamed. "Hello! HELLO! I am the one who is supposed to be in DENIAL not you!"

"I am not in denial." She said defiantly.

"How do you know? If you are in denial, you wouldn't know."

Susan was getting mad and holding it all in.

"I am the therapist here."

"So what does that make you? God?"

She stopped. Looked down and then up.

"Ken, I don't know if I am the right therapist for you. Why don't we do this? Why don't you go home and think about it, and then call me if you think I am the right therapist for you, and we will go from there."

"BUT I NEED HELP NOW! I have friggin BABY KEN in my hip! And I feel like there are hands on my throat!

"You don't have to be so dramatic!"

"But this is DRAMATIC, GOD DAMNIT! This is insane! It's nuts. What's happening to me?"

Susan looked me right in the eye.

"Go home. Think about things. And then call me if you wish."

She turned to her desk, ignoring me.

Now I have had abandonment issues in the past, BUT WHAT DO YOU DO WHEN YOUR THERAPIST ABANDONS YOU?

"Susan?"

No answer.

Susan?

No answer.

Oh boy…so not fun…

I felt a tightness in my throat… but it wasn't my imaginary strangler coming back for more fun.

It was fear. Utter gut-wrenching fear.

Am I going crazy? Am I that by-product of my late father. I am so angry! Am I becoming him?

No. No. I can't go there.

Flashback: I am auditioning for a college acting scholarship at Adelphi University in 1976. I was asked to do an improv exercise with some other actors where I was to play a baby dinosaur. If I was going to win this thing I had to go for it like I never went for anything in my life. The improv began. I was a hungry little dinosaur and I wanted my food. I really wanted my food, but the other dinosaurs didn't want me to eat. So I got mad, real mad, so frigging mad, my face curled, my voice rasped, and I transformed so much so I actually scared the other actors.

I left thinking I aced the scholarship.

Later, I heard from my girlfriend (who was on the scholarship board) that I was rejected.
They said I was TOO ANGRY, and that I was potentially dangerous to others and no way on earth would they ever give me the scholarship or even want me on campus.

And now it was 25 years later, and the DINOSAUR was back. Something ANGRY was coming out of me, hurting me and striking out at others. And I felt like I couldn't stop it.

I have to keep it in! I have to keep it in!

I HAVE TO KEEP IT IN!

Oh God, please…

CHAPTER FIFTEEN

I found myself in the pizza parlor in the shopping center in Goldens Bridge, NY. I was feeling really anxious, crazy anxious, so almost crazy, like things were happening in my body and I couldn't stop them. I felt the hands on my neck and an occasional imaginary punch on my back. And my head was starting to shake..

...shake in public.

Man, I had to stop this. I had to.

I ordered two large slices with Broccoli Rabe and a Coke and I ate as fast as I could. I felt like I was going to throw up and hyperventilate at the same time. And it wasn't from the Garlic in the Broccoli Rabe. It was from the People, the People in my Hips.

"Oh hell, I was coming undone. The pizza wasn't working, it wasn't grounding me, it wasn't helping me. Oh God please, what is going on?"

I left and went out to the parking lot outside.

I frantically called my friend Joanna seeking her help.

"Hi Joanna! Um, uh something is happening to me. Something crazy. Something I can't explain. I think…… I need some help."

I was crying.

"It's OK. What is happening?" She spoke softly from her end of the line.

"Something is happening to me. I don't know what. I have People. People in my Hips. It is a long story."

"I don't understand what you mean, but I am here to help if you need me."

"No, no, I am fine. I just need someone, a therapist, or a witch doctor or something to help me. You know someone, don't you?"

"Yes, I do. Let me get the number of my therapist. She does bodywork and more. Hold on, I am here for you." She got off the phone.

I started to feel the hands on my throat. I shook my head violently side to side. A couple of teenagers coming out of Baskin Robbins gave me a funny look.

Joanna is one of my oldest friends and a wealth of information when it comes to alternate therapies. She was back on the phone with her therapist's information.

"Her name is Karen Judge. She works out of her house in the suburbs of New Haven, Connecticut. You are going to be OK, Ken. You are going to be OK."

CHAPTER SIXTEEN

It was dark. I was lying on an old mattress in the basement of a house in the suburbs of New Haven. Karen Judge, a 60 year old hippy bodywork therapist was sitting on the floor by me with her hand on my chest right over over my heart.

My teeth were chattering, my left leg was shaking. My eyes were closed. I could hear her whispering softly:

"Know that you are safe. We are going to go back. Back to a time when all this happened when the little boy inside was safe, safe to play, safe to be alive. Let's go back. I'm here. It's safe, Ken, it's safe.

Suddenly the room started to spin. My left leg started to kick violently. My hands leaped from the mattress.

"Oh Shit! Here we go again!"

I was in my bedroom. I was young, something was happening. My Dad was yelling. Throwing things, threatening. My Dad was being CRAZY! I was so so scared. And I was HURT. Something happened! Something happened! What happened? What the hell happened? What was going on? Dad, please no…what are you going to do?

My body started to vibrate and jump like someone speaking in tongues at a revival church meeting.
I wailed, I wailed, I wailed in pain! I felt like my teeth would break from the intense chattering, and I felt like my head was ready to pop right off my neck.

I felt like I was going to die.

No, I don't want to die, not now, not now please!!

Oh my God, what was happening?

"I think your child needs some help." Karen whispered. "Can you give your child something to protect him? What can you give him? How can you help him?"
I was so confused and scared. I started a yoga teacher training program and now I am lying on an old mattress in some New Age hippy therapist's basement channelling in some lost traumatic event where I was brutally beaten by my late father. And now, this New Age hippy was asking me to GIVE something to my child self to protect my child self?
This is nuts, crazy. What the hell am I doing here?
And I felt so scared. A 45 year old man still in fear for his life, 40 years later….

Oh God, no!

I grew up on Comic books. Batman, Superman, Green Lantern and the Justice League were my heroes and because of that I believe in truth, justice and good triumphing over evil. So then and there in my post traumatic wacked-out-of-my-mind state, I decided to give my child self **ALL THE POWERS OF ALL THE SUPERHEROES IN THE WORLD!** I gave him the strength of Superman, the intellect of Batman, the power ring of Green Lantern and the combined powers of the Justice league and I we my child self Baby Ken or whatever the hell was in me FOUGHT BACK!

TAKE THAT YOU GOD DAMN MOTHER FUCKER!

HOW DARE YOU HURT ME! NEVER AGAIN!
DO YOU HEAR ME? GOD DAMN IT! NEVER AGAIN!

NEVER AGAIN!!!!!!

When I finished, I lay there totally spent as if I had just had sex with the entire Dallas Cowboy Cheerleading Squad.

TWICE.

There was no more shaking. No more teeth chattering. Something had shifted. My body was grounded.

I paid Karen Judge a hundred bucks and I was on my way, still scared, confused but grounded, very grounded, extremely grounded.

But as I lay in bed that night, I thought to myself. "What else have I forgotten?"

And I felt an icy shiver in my right hip…..

CHAPTER SEVENTEEN

OK, now we are going to get into some DARK STUFF.

Now I don't really like DARK STUFF. I would rather not talk about it. But DARK STUFF is real. We can process away negative emotions, but one can't process away DARK STUFF.

DARK STUFF is DARK STUFF and that is the be all end of it all.

But we don't have to give it power.

While Karen Judge was taking me back into my past with her HANDS ON therapy. I learned something.

I don't really know if it is true, but…it could be.

When the "People in my Hips" started going crazy in me, I filmed as much of the process as was humanly possible. I filmed video journal sessions, Yoga sessions and psychotherapy sessions.

I also filmed my session with Karen Judge. I have reviewed it again and again, for what I discovered was unfathomable.

Karen, at one point took her hands off my heart and had worked down my body to my right lower leg.

I was told by my parents that when I was very young, my right tibia (lower leg) was deformed, and it had to be broken to be put back into place.

Was that true? Sounds like a rational thing, huh?

But in my session with Karen Judge, when she touched my right leg, I remembered my father breaking it.

That's fucked up.

Did my crazy-at-the-time father BREAK my leg in a fit of unfettered rage?

I don't really know, but my body told me something.

What I do know is, that NOW, 40 plus years later, I forgive my father for ALL of his atrocities. It doesn't mean I condone his actions. It means I simply forgive him, and LOVE him forever with all of my being.

Walking back into and looking at my "People in my Hips" journey has been mind-boggling for me. I am seeing the totality of my life and my journey here thus far in a new light. So many of us are trapped by, crazy angry about, and just plain programmed by our messed up pasts, so much so that we are unable to show up in the present as who WE REALLY ARE.

The past is over.

It is no one's fault.

We can't change it.

It's done.

But today, now, we have the power and awareness to change ourselves, and in that transformation of self, we have the ability to literally change the world and our future.

CHAPTER EIGHTEEN

The next day after my superhero adventure with Karen Judge, I awoke and my hip was really tight but there was no random teeth chattering, no hands on my neck, and no imaginary blows to my back. Whatever Karen Judge had done with me on that mattress had grounded me, somehow resolving the Post Traumatic Stress/TIME TRAVEL that I had been experiencing.

But as I got out of bed, I stretched my hip….
   …And I started to shake a bit.

"BABY KEN, are you still there?"

Nothing.

And then WHAM, my head quickly shook side to side.

"He is still here. DAMN, I'm not cured," I moaned to myself, "but at least now I can function again."

Somehow I had put the lid on Pandora's Box, but I still had to deal with BABY KEN and the demons inside.

Now the thought that my father had actually broken my leg was still reverberating through my psyche.

WHAT AM SUPPOSED TO DO WITH THAT?

And who the hell knows if that was even true?

When someone is the victim of trauma, it is like the hard disk on their internal computer is smashed. When they go to retrieve data/memories, the connections are all messed up, so incomplete memories often appear or data that seems like it might be real shows up in the memory search engine. I had been remembering a myriad of CRAZY memories during Yoga and then, in daily life, but was what I was remembering real, or was it a misplaced memory file?

Contrary to POPULAR BELIEF, remembering traumatic events is not necessarily the path to healing trauma. Keeping memories, experiences and various parts of yourself, firmly associated in my past is a much better way to go. I was hoping that if I remembered the "lost" events I would be healed. Far from it. But I continued trying to remember these events, even by going back to places where I felt something happened to unearth memories thinking that that was the solution. Obviously,

I had forgotten things. DARK STUFF. And in my naivete, I decided that I would do what it takes to uncover and recover my past.

I could function more or less. I just had a displaced "child-self" by the name of Baby Ken living in my hips who was trying to tell me things, things which I THINK I had forgotten.

So frigging bizarre, huh?

I would be feeling fine and then all of a sudden I would feel a sharp pain in my hip flexor, sometimes seeing a vague image of the woods or of a wooden porch or of a bedroom, and then I would be a mess for days. Sometimes, working privately with Douglass doing yoga would help, but at other times, it would make my condition worse. I would stretch with a strap, go running, hang upside down from my feet, or soak for hours in a hot tub, and nothing would shift. And I would cry, random crying unconnected to a specific event, all the while pretending to friends, family, clients and students that I was OK.

I was definitely not OK. I needed to know what happened. What I had forgotten...

I called up my 73 year old mother and asked her if I could interview her about our family history. I told her that she knew things that none of us knew and that it needed to be documented on video, when the truth of the matter was, I needed a way to ask her some pointed questions about my childhood so I could figure out how to get the people out of my hips. I just couldn't tell her the truth of what was going on with me and my SPLIT. She wouldn't and couldn't understand.

I am not proud of the fact that I lied to my mother. I know there is no excuse, but I was scared and really confused about what was happening to me. And I didn't want to FREAK her out.

I still haven't told my mother about my real reason for our video interview. I don't think I ever will.

She was so thrilled to talk about her past, her parents and their history and it made her feel special, except when I asked questions about DAD. When the subject of Dad came up, things changed....

I have the two hour interview. I have never gone through the footage since that day. During the interview, I know there was one very interesting moment when she talked about Dad and shared something at the time that I thought profound, but for the life of me, even today, I can't remember it.

Is this "present day" loss of memory? Or is it my unconscious mind trying to protect me?

Sometimes, it is better not to know.

CHAPTER NINETEEN

So I was a mess. A big mess. I wasn't bouncing around in my daily life but it was still showing up in yoga and my left hip was so so tight, and…. it would "talk" to me.

When I say "talk" to me, literally, I would hear in my head "No." Or my hip would shake my head side to side to say "No." The hip talking to me thing was really weird. I mean really weird. But at least I could function, and go about my daily business. It was at night, and during my daily yoga practice where things would get scary. Sometimes I would wake up in excruciating pain, at other times, I would just feel a burning pain in my lower back, causing all the muscles there to be tight. And sometimes, I would just wake up knowing SOMETHING was wrong.

I called my sister again for a therapist referral, and she actually got back to me.

The therapist she referred me to was Katherine Foolmacher. She was a big wig therapist living in Putnam County. I called her and set up an appointment for that week.

Katherine's office was in her house, a very scary house in the boondocks of Putnam County, right above the Westchester border.

It was the like the ADDAM'S FAMILY HOUSE. I am not kidding. I parked my Green Honda Civic in her driveway and walked up a stone path to her front door and I entered into a small foyer which was empty except for a small wooden bench. There was a sign on the bench which read:

"Please sit. I will come and get you when I am ready."

I WILL COME AND GET YOU WHEN I AM READY?

This was NOT promising. I sat down, nervous about the upcoming session. A moment later, the door to the "therapy room" opened and a strange little old gray haired lady in her early 70's with a big witches wart on her nose appeared in the doorway.

I introduced myself and entered.

Her office was a mess. Magazines were piled left and right and the whole place was generally dusty and creepy. Really dusty and creepy. Kathryn sat behind her desk and gazed at me with a gentle smile.

"I am Katherine Foolmacher." She said calmly. "And what brings you here?"

And so I began telling my story. From my first Yoga cry to my inner child superhero adventure with Karen Judge I talked non-stop for about 35 minutes. Katherine listened intently.

"So that's it. And here I am." I finished.

Katherine pause. Scratched her long nose and then said, "That is some story."

"It certainly is." I replied.

Suddenly, she got strangely serious and said. "Do you know what I would like to do?"

I shook my head no.

"I would like to take all the abusive parents in the world and sit them in a circle."

"Uh huh?" I whispered.

"And I would have them all turn to the right."

"Yeah?"

"And I would have them all take their right hand and make a fist." She was very serious now.

"Uh huh?…" I murmured.

"And then WHAM! Punch the person in front of them!" She laughed fiendishly.

"Wow."

I was in shock. This was therapy?

"What would happen if they got a little of their own medicine?" she continued. "That would fix em. Yes, we will take all the abusive parents in the world and have them punch each other. It would be a better world. That would fix things."

She was advocating abuse to eliminate abuse. Something was seriously wrong here.

"So what can I do? I mean for my hip and all this madness." I asked.

"Well I don't think we can organize a group punch right away, so I guess you will have to come here and we can talk about it."

"What?"

"Come here and we can talk about it." Katherine repeated.

"But what can I do about the shaking?"

"I don't know. What do you think?"

"I don't know. I am here to get help."

Katherine smiled, a creepy smile.

"And I am here to help you help yourself. Those nasty parents… they could really use a good right hook to the jaw. " She giggled and then continued. "We are coming to the end of our session. Before we finish, is there anything that you would like to complete on?"

"No, I'm fine."

We made an appointment for another session and I left, knowing that I would never return.

That'll fix her.

CHAPTER TWENTY

After my adventure with Katherine Foolmacher,
I decided to get myself checked out physically. Maybe
this was a neurological condition that caused this child
self to talk with me.

What? A neurological problem?
That causes a psychotic break?

This was the crazy way I was thinking.

So I made an appointment with a Neurologist in Mt.
Kisco. When I arrived my hip/child self was dormant,
almost not there, almost as if that part of me did not want
to be discovered or uncovered. The doctor, I forget his
name, was a charming guy, early forties, personable, with
a great bed side manner. He introduced himself, and
asked me why I was there.

"Well, I am having some problems with my hip from
Yoga and I shake sometimes."

"What do you mean by shake?" he asked.

"I uh, well sometimes, my uh, well my head goes side to side and my hip cramps up." I was feeling almost embarrassed.

"O....K...., well, let me test you out and we'll see what we find."

He did a series of neurological tests, and I responded appropriately. No bouncing. No crying. No nothing.

Baby Ken, where are you when I need you?

When he finished the tests, he turned to me and said, "Well, you seem fine to me."

And I was. Baby Ken was asleep or hiding. He was so willing to come out on camera, but with strangers, no way. Curious, huh?

As I was driving home, I could feel he was back. My left hip tingled, just a bit, like he was giggling....or crying.

I came home, built a fire in the fireplace, and did my nightly yoga, bouncing a bit and feeling vaguely sad.

What was the solution? What the hell was my path? There was this "energy" in me which did not want to dissipate. And each day, it would show up in some odd way - hip cramping, weird random feelings, and now, I was starting to get weird bizarre behaviors. All of a sudden, I couldn't sit on a train, or in a restaurant with a male sitting behind me. It made me ....uncomfortable.

And I knew the feeling was OLD, but still I honored my
OLD feeling and always arranged my seating accordingly.

It was early November. I was meeting with Douglass
at a rental room studio on 72nd St. My hip was tight, and
I was feeling "melancholy" and I knew it was not
"PRESENT-BASED."

We began our Yoga, and immediately I started to
bounce and sob. Douglass, by this time was used to it, so
he just led me through the paces directing me into
various yoga asanas. We were doing a Cat/Downward
Dog sequence when it hit me.

"Douglass, I am going to do Yoga with Baby Ken."

He looked at me softly and replied " Let's go for it."

"I am always feeling like that part of me is not
connected but what if we were to do yoga together?"

"OK, Ken, let's find out."

Douglass then led me through a series of floor yoga
asanas. When the shaking began, I would consciously
take an image of myself as a child and merge it in my
mind with my visual representation of my body. At first
nothing happened, but after about 10 minutes, the
shaking slowed.

"Something's happening, Douglass."

"I can see that."

We continued. As we moved into a new stretch, I would take that image of my child, merge with my visual representation of my body, and my body would open up, open up rather drastically, with no shaking at all and all of a sudden my flexibility increased by upwards of 30%. It was uncanny! It was almost as if my visual representation of my body, was limiting my flexibility, and as I "messed with" that visual representational image by merging BABY KEN into the image, I stretched deeper than I had ever stretched before.

I started to laugh.

"Do you see what is going on here?"

"It's amazing, Ken. Just amazing."

All of a sudden, I was laughing as I did yoga, almost laughing as a child laughs, and as I laughed and pulled Baby Ken metaphysically in my body into my Yoga, my body opened up.

When we finished I felt like a million tax free bucks. I had never felt so open, so alive.

Centered and IN my body.

Yoga means to YOKE, to bring together. Somehow in this process, I brought Baby Ken into alignment.

For two weeks, I felt utterly amazing, like I was totally cured.

And then, Thanksgiving week arrived, and with it a belly full of family "stuff"ing. I cramped up two days before the holiday, and I ended up spending the day by myself...in fear...

...in fear of what?

There was something to learn here.

Why did the metaphysical yoga with Baby Ken seem to resolve things?

And now, why was it back?

CHAPTER
TWENTY-ONE

This was going to be scary.

Christmas.

I so didn't want to have my family know about my condition, and I was terrified my "stuff' would come up on Christmas eve, and all of a sudden, there would be a 6th child sitting at the Christmas Eve dinner table - BABY KEN. Yes, I can make light of all this now, but I was so damned scared, and I didn't really know what it was deep inside me that was scaring me so badly. ….but he/she/it was one nasty mother-F-er.

I felt like a leper. I was diseased somehow. I was having this "energy imbalance" or "nervous breakdown" whatever you would like to call it, but it was odd, strange, weird, and if I talked about it, no one would understand…so it became THE TIGHT HIP again. That is what I would tell my family and friends if I was buckled over in pain and starting to shake. I would say that I have a tight hip.

Oh jeez…

I didn't Christmas shop for I had no "significant other" and the only one I had to buy for was my mother and every year I gave her a hundred dollar Macy's gift card so I was done, plus, wandering around crowded stores wasn't good for my condition. It made me real paranoid.

Now paranoid was not me. That is not who I believed I was, but it was what I was experiencing at times, in restaurants or crowded places. All of a sudden, these places weren't safe. I knew it was just old "stuff" coming out of my hips, but I honored it if I could. I wasn't about to do anything to cause this "stuff" to come up. I've been there, done that and got the bouncing yoga to prove it.

The Christmas season was suddenly cold, dark, lonely… and…

NO. I vowed to myself I would not go there.

No matter what I would feel this holiday I would not believe the feelings. They were old and I knew they were old. And they weren't real. And I was going to find some way to get through this, and once through, I would help other people get through.

That was my thinking. That was how I kept upbeat. This was my story, the unbelievable story of a lifetime, and I was in the middle of it, hoping to somehow get to the last page where everything is A.O.K. and hunky-dory again.

Little did I know that I was writing WAR AND PEACE.

But the task before me was Christmas. Thanksgiving had brought my "Stuff" back after I "Yoga-cized" it out of me with BABY KEN. Since Thanksgiving, I had tried many times to take BABY KEN to the yoga mat with me, but strangely, he wasn't interested. The holidays were somehow unnerving. Thanksgiving brought it up again. Christmas could push me into the Abyss.

That place of no return.

where the Dark Man triumphs,

...and that lost little child never stops crying.

"God rest ye, Merry Gentlemen, let nothing you dismay..."

Oh hell...

CHAPTER
TWENTY-TWO

Christmas traditionally is a time for families to get together, celebrate, exchange presents and have a Merry good time.

I was terrified.

There was something inside me. Something causing me to cramp up. Something causing me to shake, causing me to be bizarrely paranoid, and something TALKING to me...

And it wasn't saying "Merry Christmas to all and to all a good night!"

No, it certainly wasn't.

Now truth be told, I really wasn't terrified. The part of me, that Baby Ken part of me, was terrified, frightened, ready to run, or just plain frozen by the Holiday chill, the Holiday fear. Another part of me, was fascinated.

I went through my days before Xmas in solitude. I worked, pretending I was Ok, then I would come home, build a fire in the fireplace, do my daily yoga practice where I would bounce around and then I would make a hot bath and just sit in the tub. Sometimes I would spontaneously break into tears, other times I would just sit numbly hot in the tub, trying not to think, yet so curiously confused about what was happening in my body.

Something about the holiday was bringing it up, or was it the cold? Did something happen to me in the cold?

As I write this tonight, I remember a memory I remembered back then which I think I have somehow tucked away.

We used to go ice skating down by the Mill Pond in Yorktown Heights when I was young. I wasn't a good skater but I loved being down on the ice at night. It was cool, almost magical, skating on the pond under the winter stars. The air was crisp and I felt so alive. We would put on our skates down by the PINE FOREST there....

"NO NO NO NO NO! Please I don't want to know. NO not now! Not now, it's over! It's over!"

On one wintry night, as I sat in a hot bathtub, being numb, something hit me, no not physically, just a thought, a memory, but the memory was so thick with pain and poison that my body started to shiver as I lay in the hot soapy water.

It was THE PINE FOREST. Something happened to me by pine trees. Something so not good, so not fun, so mind numbingly nasty that I could barely make it out on the outer edges of my consciousness. And it wasn't just the near the pine trees, it was all through the woods there.

I was running, frightened, terrified …

...of the DARK MAN.

I wept, while I shivered in the hot soapy brine.

What exactly happened, I couldn't discern. But it was clear something did happen. Something horrific. Something dark.

Something EVIL.

Wow! How's that for a Christmas present?

…and this was just the beginning of my People in my Hips Yuletide celebration.

CHAPTER TWENTY-THREE

Every year my family spends Christmas Eve at my mother's house. It not much of an event for we don't exchange gifts (except for the Macy's gift card I always get my mother) and there is no special dinner there. My Mom usually just puts out cold cuts and rolls - but that Xmas, my first "People in my Hips" Christmas was DANGEROUS. Why it was DANGEROUS I have no idea, but I knew it would be - the past, my dark past was so connected to the present then. I was fearful as to what might happen on that oh so special and SILENT NIGHT.

I wandered into Macy's in the Jefferson Valley shopping mall. It was two hours before I was to arrive at my mother's house three miles away. I needed to get her gift card before Macy's closed, and I needed to walk and walk and walk.

It was upon me, the fear, the anxiety, I didn't know what it was but it was with me.

I picked out a card and told the cashier I needed $100 on it and that it was for my mother. I always talk too much to cashiers. I didn't need to talk. I needed to move. I bought it and rushed out.

I drove down to Barnes and Noble. I would look at books and eat a big chocolate chip cookie. Maybe it would go away. I could distract it and stuff it down with sugar. I didn't want to bring it with me to Mom's, I mean I was bringing a hundred dollar gift card. That was enough. I didn't need to bring...

... THE FEAR.

"This is old stuff. This is not the present moment. This is coming out of my hips!"

Books. Books. Books.

"Oh no, not the self help section. No, Ken distract yourself, distract yourself!!!"

Books on Post Traumatic Stress Disorder - only one, but yes, my symptoms are sort of the same, but I didn't go to war or get in a car accident. Or did I?

"Ken GO AND EAT THE COOKIE! GO AND EAT THAT GOD DAMMED SO DELICIOUSLY SWEET COOKIE. IT WILL SAVE YOU SAVE YOU, SAVE YOU FROM THE FEAR!!!!!"

I got a cookie. And a latte with chocolate syrup in it. I sat...waited...chewed slowly.

I was scared, but I knew it was from THE PAST. It was old yet it felt so real.

It was time to go to Mom's.

Another cookie? No.

Suck it up, Ken. Suck it up.

It is time to pretend.
Pretend that everything is OK.

As I drove up the Taconic State Parkway to Mom's for Christmas eve, I was beyond nervous. It was like I was returning to the scene of a crime.

Traditionally, when I visited Mom on the Holidays, the entire evening, I would go in and out of the refrigerator and pick at whatever was inside. I could always find Breyer's Light and Lively Butter Pecan Ice Milk. Why my mother ate this I have no idea, but when I arrived, almost immediately, I would pick and pick and pick at this hideous frozen delight.

Obviously, my picking was a way to stave off the bad feelings that had always been under my skin. This time, those feelings, were above ground, hanging out on my shoulder like a dead squid, or hiding like a leech on my neck, ready to scream BLOODY MURDER at any second, at any second.

DAMN, I was so scared. My secret could be revealed. That I am like her x-husband. The man she watched check himself into St. Vincent's Psychiatric Hospital in Harrison, NY in the late 1960's where he was to receive SHOCK THERAPY.

"I'm BACK!! HERE'S HENRY!"

My father was dead, yet I felt like I was that crazy man returning to his family. The crazy guy who couldn't control his feelings. The Crazy-Oh-So Loving-After-He-Was-Oh-So-Bad father returning to the fold.

I parked my Green Honda Civic in front. I couldn't park in the driveway. What if I got blocked in? What if I couldn't escape? What if my feelings took over and they all saw how fucked up and scared I was....

I needed an escape route.

As I walked down the cement walkway to the front door to Mom's Christmas Paradise, my head started to twitch side to side.

STOP IT! STOP IT! NOT NOW.

I rang the doorbell.

My eyes filled with ALMOST TEARS.

The door opened. Mom. She looked good.

The whole crew was there - my step-father Paul, my brother Mike, my sister Margie, my sister Cathy and Paul's very strange son, Paul with his wife, Betty.

It was party time.

I stepped in greeted everyone. All was fine.

DON'T STAY LONG, KEN. IT IS NOT SAFE!
DON'T LINGER!

The Christmas Eve table was set. Paper plates with plastic utensils, macaroni salad, sweet gerkins, mustard, Miracle whip, buns and cold cuts.

(Where the hell are the SEVEN FISHES? My mother, God love her, just doesn't know from food.)

I walked to the refrigerator and opened the freezer and pulled out the Breyer's Butter Pecan. Here we go!

It was nice to see everyone… but underneath it all, in me, there was this little voice, maybe Baby Ken, I am not sure, but he/she/it kept repeating from some dark corner of my mind

"YOU BETTER GET OUT OF HERE! Don't linger.
They'll know!"

What will they know? THAT I AM GOING CRAZY? That I can't control my body at times, and that SOME KID PART OF ME TALKS TO ME ALL THE TIME?

Or was it something else that they might find out about? Something else many many many years ago that I had to keep a secret, and if I didn't, something something

something so bad so heinous so horrific would have happened to me, and to, maybe, everyone that I loved….

I sat with Step-Father Paul on the couch. An old 1950's war movie was playing on the TV. Paul wasn't much of a talker, a brave and wonderful man, but not much of a talker and at the time, neither was I, so I just stared at the TV pretending to be interested.

POTATO CHIPS and DIP. EAT IT KEN. NOW. YOU WILL FEEL BETTER.

My Brother Mike came over. We chatted. He kinda half-knew what was going on with me, but not really, but I could tell he was concerned. He is an awesome man. I am blessed to have him as a brother. I told him I was fine. Good. All good.

GET OUT OF HERE! NOW! GET OUT! SOMEONE IS COMING and it is NOT ST. NICK!

Mom sat next to Mike and started complaining about her camera which wasn't working right. Mike tried to help.

I got up and went to the refrigerator. I needed more BUTTER PECAN. BREYER's BUTTER PECAN ICE MILK - LOW IN FAT, HIGH IN SUGAR. The sugar will save me.

Time for dinner, or cold cuts, or Christmas Eve snack or whatever you want to call it. I sat down with a Ginger ale. My sister Margie asked my how I was doing?

"I am fine. All good. Just good."

Get some cold cuts now and shove them down your throat, Ken. Eat. Eat. STUFF IT DOWN.

I started to move funny. My hands were filled with energy. I was unsettled.

BUT DON'T LET THEM SEE. DON'T LET THEM SEE. YOU'RE NOT CRAZY!

Dinner's over. Bad Entemann's Chocolate Cake for desert. I had three pieces. I just kept picking.

Go Go Go Go Go GET THE FUCK OUT OF HERE! GO GO GO!!!

"MOM, I gotta go. Here's a present for you. Nothing new, but I think you will like it.

"Oh my Macy's card. Thank you. HOW DID YOU KNOW?" she said with a wink.

"You're easy."

THE FEELING was coming upon me. That scared little boy feeling. That **I-don't-have-any-control-here** feeling. Oh shit, I have to get out now.

"Ok, it was great seeing you all. Love you. Merry Christmas!"

I closed the front door behind me and ran to my car. I zigged quickly down the path to my car.

It was up. It was happening.
THE FEELING was upon….me.

I quickly climbed into my Green Honda Civic and my body started to fling itself about the car like I was on a enclosed trampoline. As I bounced around, my head shook violently from side to side. It was insane. Nuts. Crazy. What was going on in me! *HELP ME PLEASE! MOMMY, HELP ME PLEASE! MOMMY MOMMY PLEEEEEEEEEEEEEEEZE!*

The bouncing subsided. I sat there in the freezing cold car stunned, weeping softly.

All I wanted for Christmas was my life back…

CHAPTER
TWENTY-FOUR

Gil Arati, BODY PSYCHOLOGIST, was a tall, wiry, dark-haired man, with a dark olive complexion. He introduced himself and walked me into his large office/studio that had views looking out over northern Manhattan. I was referred to him by a dancer friend of mine. This was the Big City bodywork dude who was going to cure me.

"Let's start over here on the mat." Gill said with a sly smile. "So you say you are experiencing a lot of energy in your body.

"I'll say."

All of a sudden my head twitched side to side. There was something about him that was unsettling, odd. My body didn't like him. He was creeping me out.

He looked at me strangely and said, "Ok lets try a roll down. Just drop your chin to your chest and roll down. I want to see what is going on here."

I rolled my spine down slowly. As I got to halfway, my body suddenly shook up and down and I started to hyperventilate slightly.

Baby Ken was in the room.

"HMMMM…." Gil sighed. "When you reach the bottom, roll up very very slowly."

I reached the floor and then I slowly rolled up. As I reached that same point in the middle of my spine, I started to bounce again, this time more violently.

"Huh?" Gil said. "Now roll up all the way and then down again."

I rolled and then started rolling down again. This time at that same point in my spine my head started to shake violently side to side like something out of a cartoon.

"Continue down and then roll up again. There's a lot of energy here. Lots of energy."

Gil seemed perplexed. He was creeping me out.

"Yes, there is…." I replied. "Lots of energy and this is only about 5 on a scale of 1 to 10.

"And you say this started from Yoga?" he questioned.

"Yeah. Yoga. Do you believe it? Next time I need stress relief I'll work more.

"Can you roll down again?"

"Sure." This time my entire body bounced as if I was on a bouncing trampoline in an earthquake.

"I've never seen this." Gil said semi-shocked.

"This is nothing. You should see me on a good day."

"Really?" He was totally perplexed. "Ok roll up. Let's have a seat."

I sat on a small black couch off from the matted area. He sat across from me on another small black couch.

"So have you ever considered neuroleptic drugs?" he asked softly.

What the hell was he talking about? I am not crazy. I am not my father. There will be no shock therapy on my watch. No F-ing way.

"No. Neuroleptic Drugs shrink the brains of monkeys." I replied. "My brain is small enough now."

"Uh huh. Hmmmm." He stared at me again for another long uncomfortable moment. "What is that I see in your eyes? Is it anger?"

WHAT THE HELL IS HE TALKING ABOUT?

"No, there is no anger in my eyes. I have people in my hips." I replied defiantly.

He stared.

"It seems like there is something behind your eyes that is angry. What is it?"

WHAT THE HELL IS HE TALKING ABOUT?

"There is nothing angry behind my eyes." I whispered hoarsely. "Behind my eyes is my shrunken Monkey brain."

"That's funny." He laughed.

"I'm being serious." I stared at him.

He looked down and then looked up again into my eyes. I stared back.

"I see you are…very serious."

He stared even deeper into my eyes. My eyes locked back in the ultimate status battle. I would not look away. There was no ANGER in here. No F-ing Anger!

"I still say I see something behind your eyes."

"Well, you must be hallucinating?" I fired back. "Maybe you should prescribe yourself some neuroleptics."

He smiled again oh-so slyly.

"Maybe I should."

There was a long pregnant pause.

"So can you help me?" I asked.

He stared. Paused, and then spoke.

"I think I can." He paused again, and then smiling again oh-so slyly… "But it is going to require us to get together and do some very challenging work."

"I'm up for it. Are you?" I smiled back.

"I see anger in there."

WOULD YOU JUST GET OFF THIS!

"I have no anger in my eyes. If there is anger anywhere, it is in my hips. I have god-damn fucking people in my hips, but there is no, I repeat no, anger in my eyes."

He stared, and then paused for about twenty seconds and said, "I see. So why don't we set up a time for our first real session and we will take it from there?"

I was crazy mad. I came for his help to get this stuff out of my hips and here he is accusing me of having ANGER in my eyes. If there was any anger in my eyes it was created by our interaction.

"Sure. Let's set up a session."

So we made an appointment for the next week, but I called him the next day.... It went like this:

MESSAGE MACHINE: Hello, this is Gil Aratz. Please leave a message when you hear the tone.

"Hi Gil this is Ken Wolf. I am calling today cancel our appointment."

Tears started to arise in me, a waterfall of emotion...

"I want to be very clear with you. There is no anger in my eyes. There is no anger in my eyes."

THAT GOD-DAMNED BASTARD.

"Someone once said that 'The eyes are the windows to the soul.'"

My body started to shake as salty tears of forgotten pain fell on the phone.

"Well, my soul is not angry. My soul is not angry! My soul is loving and strong. It is the one part of me that has kept me going, kept me alive through this process of trying to cure myself."

My whole body started to tremble.

"My soul is all I have. And it is not angry. It is my best and truest friend. So I am canceling our session next week and forever. What you saw in my eyes must have been your own reflection."

I hung up slowly.

I could sense a presence in my left hip, scared, so so scared, ...Baby Ken.

And in my right hip, another presence, a foggy memory of my distant past, arising, growing somehow out of my body.

It had no name, yet I knew what it was.

It was Evil.

CHAPTER
TWENTY-FIVE

Yanni Dilosky was a TRAUMA HEALING THERAPIST
visiting from Germany. I was referred to him by one of my
Yoga teacher trainer friends. Yanni was an advocate of the
TAMING THE TIGER method developed by Peter Levine.

Now the therapeutic metaphor from The TAMING the
TIGER method was this: In nature let's say when a tiger is
chasing an antelope and the antelope manages to get
away, the antelope releases its traumatic stress by shaking
it's entire body for about 30 seconds. At the end of this
shaking session, the antelope is stress-free, in a new
moment in now with no residual fear of the tiger and it
can go about its business. Granted I was a bit skeptical
about this method, for I had already been shaking for six
months, and my TIGER still had its teeth fully embedded
in my ass and it wasn't letting go.

Yanni was staying with a fellow trauma healing
therapist in an apartment on 45th St. between Eighth and
Ninth Ave in Manhattan. This was where he did his
therapy.

It was a cold January day when I journeyed down to the Big City again to meet another variety of therapist. As always, I was nervous, and scared. What if doing this therapy with Yanni brings my stuff up and I can't get out of it. What if it takes over? How will I make a living? How will I survive? ..... And what if "Baby Ken" decides to move in?

Now that is scary.

It was an old building about halfway down 45th St. right next to Private Eyes, a gentleman's club, where strippers hang out. I never understood that gentleman's club metaphor. Private Eyes was a strip club. There was nothing gentlemanly about it.

I rang the bell for 14C and I was buzzed in. I took the elevator up.

Oh no, here we go again.

Yanni was a heavyset light-haired man with a thick German accent. He was about 28 and he was wearing a gray Led Zeppelin tee shirt and a frayed vest. He invited me in. It was a studio apartment with one large window with three panes looking north. The furniture was old, worn and there was a slight dusky smell of cigarettes.

"So I was referred to you by one of my Yoga associates. I am having strange crazy things happen in my body. I am bouncing, cramping up, and I cry a lot. It is all connected to my childhood somehow or events that I have forgotten in my childhood."

He was staring at me.

"Yes, I understand. Ve don't need to talk too much." He said flatly. "I am un student of Peter Levine, und I haf vorked with him at many of his seminars und veekend gatherings. His therapy is a little different. I am just visiting here and I am going back to Germany to vork with him for a veek long intensive.

WELL GOOD FOR YOU… I wanted to say.

"So this is vat I vant you to do." Yanni said softly in his thick German accent. "Find some space in dis room where you feel safe, and den tell me vere you vant me to be."

"What?" I was confused.

"Experience da room from a safe perspective. And tell me vere I can be dat it is safe for you."

"What?"

Yanni continued. "Are you safe un front of da vindow, or are you safe under dat table? Find out. And den tell me vere I should go - behind you, to da left to da right."

"OK."

I walked around the room trying to FEEL "vere" I was safest. It was so bizarre. I think I would have been safer down at Private Eyes getting a lap dance.

"Ok. I am pretty safe here."

"And vere shall I go?"

"You just go up over there to my right."

"Do you feel safe now?" Yanni whispered.

"Yeah, sort of."

"Now lift your arms und start moving dem in space. Vat do you sense? Vat do you feel?"

I start to move my arms around in the air. Too weird.

"I feel self-conscious and I feel like a jerk."

"Let me know if your hands tingle. Ven hands tingle often dat is a sign that trauma is being released."

"When my hands tingle?"

"Yes, dey tingle and den POOF the trauma energy is released."

"And what happens when I click my ruby slippers together 3 times?" I asked wryly.

"I don't understand."

"American Pop culture reference. A quote from THE WIZARD OF OZ."

BOOM!

ALL OF A SUDDEN THE FEELING WAS UPON ME.

Like a cobra striking it's prey **THE FEELING** was there so fast so strong so present and so past.

I started to shake a bit, and tears welled up in my eyes. I started to see vague images and I could feel a tingle in my left hip. Damn, I was scared so crazy scared again out of nowhere. The room then started to spin. Yanni stood in the corner not really looking at me but somehow listening and sensing what was going on with me. The emotions started to move and I was just standing there, not doing Yoga, not even thinking about the past but stuff memories ideas history my past my lost past my who I was that I forgot was somehow coming back in this dirty little apartment on 45th St.

"WHOA! SHIT! I am not feeling safe. Not safe at all!" I yelled.

"Vat do you see? What do you feel?" Yanni yelled back.

Oh no, here it comes!

BOOM!

"FOLLOW IT! FOLLOW IT!" Yanni screamed.

The shaking grew stronger. *Oh no not again!* And stronger. *Oh, please no, I have had enough.* My head started to jackhammer back and forth. Images came flooding into my consciousness. So weird, so bizarre. What I was seeing made no sense!

"I HAVE TO STOP!" I yelled to Yanni.

I knelt down on the floor.

"Are you alright?" Yanni whispered.

"Yes."

"Vat did you see?" Yanni asked softly.

It was too weird.

"I saw my grandfather. Only he was younger, in his thirties, dressed funny, something was happening… it was bad. How can I see my grandfather when he was in his thirties? I wasn't alive yet."

Yanni paused, thought for a moment, and then responded.

"There are more things in heaven and earth, then are dreamt in our philosophy. Sometimes memories are passed through our DNA."

Grampa was back.

And his dentures now were firmly embedded

...in my ass.

CHAPTER TWENTY-SIX

How do you live your life when at a moment's notice you start to channel in random crazy abuse propelled into the present from your past?

It was a challenge. After Yanni, I was frustrated out of my mind because our little TRAUMA HEALING ADVENTURE did nothing but bring more stuff up for me - the mystery of my Grandfather.

How could I see my Grandfather when he was in his thirties? I was far from being born. Was that a memory or a hallucination? And what could it mean? Why did I SEE that? Was it my unconscious mind telling me something or what?

I decided to bag the therapists and work with Douglass and create my own program of discovery.

No one knew what was going on with me, and the more I worked with people the more confusing it was. My answer lie in following my intuition, following my gut, for the answer to my dilemma was a dilemma, an unknown factor, a big f-ing question mark.

So I worked with Douglass, as much as possible.
My answer lie in my body. We would explore with yoga.

Now I know this sounds crazy. Technically, you could
say I had PTSD, and sort of a psychotic break (the talking
to Baby Ken part) but what if it wasn't PTSD, what if it
wasn't a psychotic break, what if it were something else?

It began in my body with yoga, and I was sure the
answer lie with my body with yoga, or at least with
bodywork.

So Douglass and I continued our work. I would cry a
lot and bounce about. Douglass would watch in quiet
amazement. We explored new ways to stretch my hips,
using ropes, blocks and various props. One time, we
hung ropes from the ceiling and hung my different limbs
off the ropes and stretched in crazy and fun ways.
I shook, and cried, and moaned and sometimes laughed
hysterically but I was determined to cure myself of this
wacky condition.

It was June, 2004. It had been almost a year living
with the people in my hips. Despite all my yoga work, the
truth of the matter was, I wasn't getting better. The People
in my Hips had taken over my life.

It was a Sunday afternoon and I was driving on my
way to Walmart in Mohegan Lake to do some shopping.
The route I took to Mohegan Lake required that I pass
through my old home town of Yorktown Heights where I

grew up. I had driven this route by myself on many occasions and there was never a problem, but this particular Sunday afternoon things were different.

As I drove down Route 202 through Yorktown, suddenly, I wasn't alone.

DON'T GO THERE! GET AWAY! Don't go there! GET AWAY!

Oh hell, it was a little voice in my head screaming at me?

DON'T GO THERE! GET AWAY! Don't go there! GET AWAY!

I quickly pulled into the Staples parking lot near where I used to live and and parked.

What the hell is going on!

My body was shaking and my head was bouncing side to side.

STAY AWAY! RUN AWAY! DON'T GO THERE!

I pushed back my seat back, lay back flat, shook and wept hysterically for 30 minutes. A little voice screaming in my ear:

Don't go there!

And it wasn't referring to WALMART.

Baby Ken was telling me not to go near my old house in Yorktown, where I lived as a child for there was DANGER there.

If I went there, I would be hurt. I would be hurt…
…by the Dark Man.

 It was forty years later.
Forty years after whatever had happened. The evil.

Forty years later and a scared little voice had somehow embodied me, and then stopped me, forcing me to cry, and shake for thirty minutes in my little green Honda Civic. The house where I grew up was only a mile away. Somehow, in some crazy way, Baby Ken, was keeping me safe.

But this was crazy scary.

A half hour later, I pulled my crying self together and drove to Walmart without further psychotic communications.

That night, I called Dr. Freud.

I was referred to Dr. Bryan Freud by a friend of Jen's at work. His real name isn't Freud - I have changed his name for Client/Doctor confidentiality. I really needed help.

Bryan Freud was about thirty-eight, well-dressed, handsome, slightly balding and extremely personable. I immediately felt at home with him. On his computer, I showed him the DVD of my first baby Ken encounter where I flew around in the chair. He had never seen anything like it. Oh boy.

I spent the rest of the session filling him in on the whole crazy evolution of THE PEOPLE IN MY HIPS. We set up an appointment for the following Friday and I left.

I walked around the corner to the Starbucks on 41st and Broadway, ordered a Grande Mocha, and found a table in the corner by the window. As I sat sipping my coffee, gazing out at the hustle and bustle of Manhattan I thought to myself, "Why me? Why did this happen to me? Out of all the people in the world, why was I cursed with People in my Hips?" There were a million stories in this naked city, and somehow for some bizarre reason I was cursed with this one. And then I thought about someday curing myself and telling this tale. Sitting there, nursing my coffee, gazing out into Times Square, I quietly wept, as a million stories danced by.

CHAPTER
TWENTY-SEVEN

During my first sessions with Dr. Freud, I was simply filling him in on the blanks, details of my story, and my family history. It felt great to talk with someone impartial about my crazy condition, but was it affecting change in me? No, I don't think so.

I had a hard time with therapy. It is not that Dr. Freud wasn't good. No, he was an extraordinary consultant and member of my "People in my Hips" team. I just couldn't understand how TALKING could free me from The People in my Hips. How could words - the expression of - and the emotions that I would be feeling in session get this crazy energy out of my hips? It didn't seem possible.

Our first sessions were interesting. Dr Freud was really good at creating rapport, and I certainly felt more or less at ease with him, but part of me was holding back.
I could feel that I wasn't really talking deep, if that makes any sense. I would joke, babble about my cramping, but I really wasn't zooming in on the issue:

WHAT THE HELL HAPPENED TO ME AS A CHILD?

So in our sessions, there was little shaking, sometimes some cramping but no bouncing up and down, and no Baby Ken. I was avoiding it all. It wasn't safe. It just wasn't safe. Was it because Dr. Freud was a man? I don't know. But I didn't feel safe. So somehow I held it all in.

Somedays I would actually leave his office and then begin to shake. So bizarre!

So, in therapy I wouldn't really talk deeply. I just touched the surface. What the heck was I doing? I was paying for this, AND I HAD TO GET THE PEOPLE OUT OF MY HIPS!

And then I had an idea. What if I could film my therapy sessions? If I could film them, I would feel safe for they would be documented, and Baby Ken loved performing for the camera - he would do it three or four times a week when I filmed myself doing my nightly Yoga practice. This could be an opening, and in some crazy way, it would be fun.

So I asked Dr. Freud if I could bring my video camera into session. He was weird about it at first but I told him I would just be filming myself, so he conceded.

I was thrilled. Who gets to film real live therapy sessions? This was amazing!

And then I thought:

"And someday, when I am cured I will show one of these clips on OPRAH!"

So at our next session, I pulled out the video camera, and miraculously,

Baby Ken appeared.

(On YouTube channel: the peopleinmyhips you will find stunning video of Baby Ken literally talking with Dr. Freud and myself in therapy. Scary and amazing.)

And so began this incredible therapeutic process. Each Friday I would meet with Douglass from 4 pm to 5 pm in a rented studio on 8th Ave where we, with Yoga would unearth memories/feelings in my body and then I was off to Dr. Freud to process it all with Baby Ken…

Now we're talking!

CHAPTER
TWENTY-EIGHT

Therapy got really painful. Not just emotionally, but physically. More times than not, my hip would literally cramp up right after working privately with Douglass on my way to see Dr. Freud. Since I started filming my therapy sessions, I think the Baby Ken part of me, got scared. Scared that he would now have to relive the horrifying experiences that he had hidden or purposefully forgotten. And to be honest, I too was getting scared. I was fascinated by the filming process, but what was coming out in therapy was absolutely nuts. It was often a BABY-KEN-LET-IT-ALL-OUT- BOUNCEFEST. My head would vibrate back and forth like a washing machine on steroids. I would suddenly cry this high pitched and bizarre cry out of nowhere and my left leg would bounce up and down constantly.

One day when I arrived at therapy, my hip was so locked up that I couldn't sit. So I stood, half-crunched in fear, trying to work it all out. Even now when I think about it, I was SOOOOOOOOOO messed up, but often in life, in order to heal, one needs to get to that totally whacked out place in order to return to normal.

"Sometimes you have to go a very long distance out of your way in order to come back correctly"
- Edward Albee -

I was in a bad place.

"You have got to help me, Dr. Freud! I'm in crazy crazy pain. I have fucking people in my hips. And it hurts. I need to get better. I gotta get better." I screamed at Dr. Freud.

"I can see you do. When did all this happen?" he responded softly.

"When did all this happen? It is happening now. I am in pain. I am being attacked from my past, and I have to get this out of me!"

"I can see you do."

"Well, help me. I need some help. Hypnotize me or something, but I have got to do something. I can't do this anymore. I can't. I just can't."

"I understand."

"I don't need your understanding I NEED YOUR HELP!" I screamed.

I was in reactive mode. I was not in the present moment. This was some old FEELING that was taking over my "now," that I was "assigning" to Dr. Freud - making him out to be the cause of my pain for he, up to this point, had been unable to cure me. (As if a therapist actually cures someone - Hello! We cure ourselves. A therapist simply leads and facilitates. We make the connections and make the choice to heal.)

"YOU HAVE GOT TO DO SOMETHING!"

"Where do you think all this stems from?" Dr. Freud asked.

"FROM MY HIPS! FROM MY HIPS!"

The people in my hips were taking over. I was somehow trapped in some old scenario, screaming for what seemed like my life. Needless to say, our session was less than productive, but that night, as I lay in bed, trying to figure out what the heck was going on, the metaphor, the old feeling, the belief system which was working on me, like a ghost of Christmas past, suddenly became clear.

I was begging DR. Freud to help me, much like I must have begged my father and/or the DARK MAN to stop hurting me. I had made some sort of mental transference associating Dr. Freud (a male authority figure) with the male abusers in my past, blaming him for my hip pain and all the other known and unknown pain from my past. The old pain appeared in my hips, I assigned it to the present moment - to Dr. Freud, and then responded as if the old feelings were real.

A feeling comes out of my body from my past. I assign it to the present moment, and respond as if it is real, using my reality (how I assigned it) to validate it.

This is very heady stuff, but can you see how we do this all the time in our lives, in relationships, at work, with our families? A feeling arises in our bodies - is triggered by some present day trigger, and then we place that feeling on our world and then justify it to be true and respond accordingly which validates it further. No wonder we have problems in our personal relationships. Often we aren't even responding to what is really happening in the present moment. We are responding to OUR PAST.

This has been one of the biggest gifts of my People in my Hips experience. I know now that my feelings are not my reality. They are just my feelings. Yes, sometimes they sneak in and try to color my reality, but for the most part now, I stand guard and challenge any feeling based reality my unconscious mind may be trying to create.

Huh?

Maybe therapy works.

CHAPTER
TWENTY-NINE

The wild part of my journey is that I was literally living with the People in my Hips for three long years. From 2003 - 2006, I had to deal with this crazy crazy whatever it was in me that would in a instant turn my life upside down.

I continued to see Douglass and Dr. Freud at least once a week. I would meet Douglass at a rented studio on 37th St. and Eighth Ave where we with Yoga would explore the very bizarre energy in my body. Some days I would show up and I would feel fine, until we began our Yoga, when all of a sudden, demons from the darkest depths of hell would suddenly manifest in my body causing me to cry and bounce around my Yoga mat.

Other times I would show up at our session a total mess. My hip may have locked up the night before in my sleep, or on the train on the way down to the city, but the pain and the unknown fear would be present in my pre-Yoga state, almost as if, whatever horrendous event my body was remembering, was literally living in my body and attacking me again. Douglass would know the moment he saw me where I was physically and emotionally and he, intuitively, would respond accordingly.

Sometimes he would just start by cradling my head in his hands and moving my head gently side to side, as my body jumped around. Other times, he would intuitively, press on points on my back as I was resting in a restorative posture. At times I would also intuitively tell him what I thought I needed - (i.e "press here" or "can we do this asana?" or "lift my left leg and shake it.") It was this wild and beautiful healing Yoga dance. Most of the time, I would feel better when we finished, but sometimes the emotion and the fear which manifested as we did Yoga would stick with me like … a scary old … friend. Yes, like a friend. I was so familiar with the fear now, we were like buddies, yet the fear had no face and no name. Did I need to see the face, hear the name in order to be cured? I had no idea.

After Yoga, I would go to Starbucks order a Mocha Latte and a large chocolate chip cookie, which I would consume ravenously, and then, I would go to Godiva next door and order a huge coconut macaroon. Somehow binging on sweets helped keep the People in my Hips at bay.

And then it was off to Dr. Freud on 42nd and Broadway, to process the Peeps in therapy, often with the help of Baby Ken.

When I look at these therapy videos, where Baby Ken and I talk with Dr. Freud, I am still amazed. It has been a little over four years since my People in my Hips adventure. But when I watch the videos, it still scares me for I never ever want to go back there. Yes, one cannot control people and situations outside of oneself, but I was unable to control people and situations INSIDE myself. All my life, I went to therapy to deal with people and things outside of myself. Here, in therapy with Dr. Freud, I was dealing with people and things INSIDE myself that I could not control. And that is damned scary.

My weekly ritual was this. Everyday when I came home from work, I would do my Yoga practice where I would bounce and cry. Sometimes I would break out the video camera and film it, other times I would just experience it.

Then I would take a hot bath for 30 minutes or so and climb into bed.

Fridays I would see Douglass and then Dr. Freud and then take the train home in time to watch Stargate SGI on TV hoping to distract myself from whatever came up in the hours before. Often, I would just cry myself to sleep, and most of the time I didn't even know what I was crying about.

What kept me going was my doggedly determined obsession with curing myself and someday helping other with this knowledge. What also kept me going was the fact that I could not live my life this way. I needed my life back. I wanted normalcy. I wanted to be in a relationship again. I wanted all of this to go away and stay away so that I could get on with my life.

But it wasn't going anywhere.

The People in my Hips had moved in.

CHAPTER THIRTY

The saving grace throughout my People in my Hips adventure was Douglass.

While I was:

cramping up,

feeling paranoid,

challenging suicidal thoughts,

channeling in a bizarre child part of me who lived in my left hip,

going to doctors,

making video journals,

getting super heroes to help me,

interviewing my mother on tape to discover the mysteries of my childhood,

dealing with the crazy energies trapped in my hips,

and hiding all this craziness from my friends and family.

Douglass was there.
Present, compassionate and strong.

We would meet at least once a week, and he would quietly watch me bounce and cry during yoga, and, like two Yoga scientists, we would experiment and explore different positions and Asanas in a quest to release the crazy unknown energy in my body. Sometimes when I was all locked up and in the thick of it my unknown physical malady, Douglass would simply manipulate my body into different Yoga stretches as I wept. And it was incredibly healing, maybe not on the physical plane, but in my emotional world, I was being divinely cared for by a man. I was savagely beaten by my father, (and maybe someone else too,) but in Yoga with Douglass I felt safe, and in that safety sparked the beginning of my greatest healing, the ability to feel safe with and cared for by a man.

I found this quote in a book of therapy short stories, and I think it applies here.

"In therapy, it's not what you do with a client , it is how you are.

It's the relationship that heals, the relationship."

Thank you, Douglass.

CHAPTER THIRTY-ONE

I walked into therapy all bent out of shape, literally. My right hip had just cramped up after my session with Douglass. I felt like I had a knife in my leg and my emotions were on edge from the feeling emanating from my hip. I silently hooked up the video camera. Dr. Freud could tell something was up.

"So?"

I sighed. I didn't want to go into it. I didn't want to talk. I was so god damned tired of talking. I wanted this STUFF out of me. It had just been going on for too long. Way to friggin' long.

"I want it out of me. Can't we do something? Like hypnosis or something - just to make it disappear, make it go away, like back into my unconscious and just stay there? Hypnotize me. Just hypnotize please..."

"We could do something like that. Do you know what timeline therapy is?"

"Yes, I'm familiar with it. Yeah, take me back, I will see it all and be healed. Let's do it." I was so done.

"I wish it was that easy, but I'm will to try it."

"Let's do it."

Dr. Freud dimmed the lights.

"Ok Ken, I want you to focus on your breathing, just allow the breath to flow in and out, and as you focus on your breathing, you can now feel your body relaxing, letting go, just allow yourself to relax, just let everything go. It is safe. It is safe here."

I didn't feel safe at all. I could feel the "Energy" swirling in my body.

Dr. Freud continued.

"As you continue to breathe and relax, you can feel your body becoming weightless, light, free, open and relaxed. You feel good. You feel safe. It is safe here. Now as you continue to breathe and relax I want you to imagine that you are floating out of your body and going up into the sky a mile or so, you can still breathe, there is plenty of air and you can float on the air. It is safe. As you look down, you can see your time line crossing right through your body one way going off into the future and the other way going back in to the past - staying way up in the sky, let yourself follow your timeline back into the past.

My body started to shake. I could feel the energy down in my hips become alive.

"You are 40, 30, 25, 20, 18,15 and when you get to the age that is important to you and to your hip, stop and let me know what you see. You can go back up into the sky at any time. At anytime you can escape if you need to..."

I needed to escape. I needed to get away. I was back there, but back there was somewhere I had never been before. It made no sense. I saw old cars, I was in Astoria where my grandmother lived but it was different. I saw old hats, old storefronts, street lamps and people, young people dressed funny like out of an old movie. I was in a bathroom, but it didn't feel like me there, it was like it was someone else but I was somehow there..., there were white tiles shaped in hexagons on the walls, the tiles were hexagons, white, brown grout.... and *NO, please NO, don't come in please don't hurt me, no no no no NOOOOOOOOO!!!!*

I know this doesn't make sense, but this is what I saw in that timeline session.

I saw Grampa Wolf, only he was young and he was hitting me and I was my father as a child. It was the 1940's before I was alive. I was being brutally beaten by my grandfather, only I was my Dad, trapped in my father's bathroom by myself in his apartment in Astoria, Queens and also on the streets there. I was seeing and experiencing what I seemed like my father's MEMORIES. Vivid and uncanny. Rich in detail and in fear. I had no knowledge Dad's family history but this crazy vision showed my grandfather brutally beating my father/me, again and again and again. Kicking, slapping, punching *OH PLEASE STOP!* and I saw my father crying, while trying so hard to protect himself from his drunken, angry father.

Suddenly I saw my father in a different light, one not condoning his brutal behavior, but through a perspective of somehow *underbtanding* it. Understanding where his brutal behavior was learned....

And somehow this memory/vision was past through my father's DNA to me.

I wept and I wept. Dr. Freud watched quietly.

Was this vision real? It would make sense with all my previous bizarre memories of my grandfather. And it felt so so real. But HOW could it be real?

Seeing my grandfather's brutal behavior towards my father made so much sense to me... but the mind works in mysterious ways. Especially with childhood trauma.

This was the question which plagued me for weeks after this session:

Was this real, or did a part of me make all this up so I could forgive my father's sins?

CHAPTER THIRTY-TWO

It was April 2004, before I went to see Dr. Freud. Before I discovered who was trapped within me. It was a Saturday afternoon, and I was driving home to my cabin in Goldens Bridge, after training some clients and I started to feel it in my right hip. Traditionally, it was in my left hip, (the "it" I am referring to is the BAD ENERGY.) I was unsettled, nervous. I would get a cup of coffee at Winston's in Armonk. The coffee would help.

I sat out in front of Winston's and sipped my coconut flavored coffee. It wasn't helping. It was getting tight, my neck was getting tight, I started to shake a bit, and I was getting paranoid.

I would run. I would run like a banshee and get this energy out of my hips. Maybe if I ran hard enough and fast enough it would go away. I threw out my coffee and went to my car.

I had been training private clients that morning so I had my workout gear on. I left my black windbreaker in the car, with my wallet. I put my keys in my pocket.

I started to walk down the block opposite Winston's. I could feel emotions rising out of my right hip. Scary feelings… and then I started to feel the burning, the burning going through my pelvis to my lower back.

OH GOD it was happening!

I started to run, first slowly and then I accelerated. My head started to shake softly side to side.

NO NOT NOW please! NOT NOW I don't want to feel it. I want you to go away! Go the HELL Away!

I burst into a sprint. Tears started to fall from my eyes, and I had no idea why. I started to yell.

"GET AWAY FROM ME! GET THE HELL AWAY FROM ME! I want you out. Get the hell out. Get out of me!"

My leg started to cramp.

NO, I am not going to let you win. I am not. NOT THIS TIME, GOD DAMNIT!

And I tried running faster.

I must have looked like a total nutcase, running down the road adjacent to Winston's and the main drag of Armonk, screaming:

"GET OUT! GOD DAMNIT, GET OUT!"

I didn't want this in me anymore. It wasn't fair. I didn't do anything! Why are you doing this to me? What did I do?

And when I look back now, I can clearly see that it was all about my unknown-lost-in-my-unconscious childhood abuse.

As a child, I experienced RANDOM childhood abuse. Unexplainable. It didn't make any sense at the time, and now, then, when I was running, when my hip was cramping, I was in effect reliving the experience. Something/someone unknown was hurting me.

Again.

I got back to my car by Winston's, limping, my face more wet from tears than sweat, and I sat on the curb with my head in my hands, my right hip wracked in pain.

The past was the present. This was not new. It was old. So very old. Forty years old. And for some reason, it decided to erupt that day, hurting me deeply, beating me silly, without remorse.

Something or someone in me...

...wanted to kill me.

CHAPTER THIRTY-THREE

Somewhere sometime in my past, there was an event, a secret trauma that I hid deep in my unconscious, and I knew The DARK MAN, the foggy, scary memory of someone from my childhood was responsible, but I couldn't remember any real details about him or the event. Whenever Dr. Freud and I would explore the Dark Man and this event with the Baby Ken part of me, I would shake violently and get really scared. It was totally crazy. Yet I knew what I was experiencing was real. And I was utterly horrified that my father might be the villain here.

On one particularly cold February Day, my hip was crazy active. Over the course of a couple of months, I had developed the unique ability to simply relax my hip and the crazy hip energy would flow and Baby Ken would appear. It was time to get answers.

"Ok, Dr. Freud," I said with pointed determination, "I am just going to release my hip. It's been real active today so somethings up."

Immediately my left leg starts to shake.

"See here he is… Wow, I think Baby Ken is on Speed today."

Baby Ken was with me, in my mind, in my body.

"Baby Ken," Dr. Freud said softly, "Can you tell me what you are feeling?"

The VOICE came from that part of me, the hurt child, the past, BABY KEN.

"It's bad."

"What's bad?"

"What he did to me?"

Dr. Freud continued.

"What did he do to you?"

My left leg bounced up and down.

"I don't know. It's a secret."

"A secret?"

Yes, a secret." Baby Ken replied. *"And I can't tell anyone."*

"Why?"

"Because he will hurt me."

"Hurt you? Who will hurt you? Your father?"

"No, someone else." Baby Ken stammered.
"Not Dad. NOT DAD. NOT Dad. Someone else.
He's going to hurt me. He's going to kill me. He'll Kill me!
He'll kill me. I have to keep it a secret! I have to! NO.
Stop! No please! I won't tell. I won't tell!

I saw myself walking up to our house in Yorktown.
I was hurt. I was hurt. Something happened.

"I can't tell anyone."

My right hand started hitting my right leg as my left
leg shook harder and harder. It was like one side of my
body started fighting with the other side. My body was
moving, shaking violently of its own accord, as I sat
watching. My body shook and I hit myself again and
again and again as I witnessed this bizarre somatic
manifestation in total disbelief. I shook faster and faster
and I hit myself harder and harder. It was nuts. It was
totally insane. What the hell was going on in my body!
My body had a mind of its own!

And then I knew.

There was another personality in my body
living in my right hip...

...it was THE DARK MAN.

CHAPTER
THIRTY-FOUR

The most frightening part of my People in my Hips experience was that I never knew when "The Peeps" would manifest. Some days I would be fine, and on others, I would be a wreck, barely even being able to walk, or just filled with OLD scary emotion from the past.

And then, some days would be LIVING HELL.

It was November. I was taking the train home from NYC after seeing Douglass and Dr. Freud. It was the 7:56 express to Goldens Bridge.

When I got on the train I knew something was up. Whatever I had opened up in Yoga with Douglass and then in therapy with Dr. Freud was starting to work on me. The train was crowded with commuters and day shoppers coming home after a long and tiresome day. Whenever I got on a train, I would immediately search for a seat with a wall behind me. Having a wall behind me felt safe. No one could hurt me from behind. At the time,

I knew it was crazy to do this, but "The Peeps" made it uncomfortable at times to sit with someone behind me, especially a man. So I wouldn't do it. I always had a train wall behind me. Unless there wasn't a safe seat available. This particular evening, that was the case. Oh hell…

So I sat by a window with a small Puerto Rican man sitting behind me. Small was good. Small may not bring the fear, plus something was brewing in me, and a big guy behind me would not work. A thirty year old woman sat down next to me with her six year old daughter. She sat her daughter between me and her. Oy!

Then behind me, I heard my worst nightmare. It was a large six foot tall business dude, booming about something stupid on his cellphone.

OH HELL NO A LOUD VOICE BEHIND ME PLEASE NOT NOW NO NOT NOW!

The train started. We began our trip through the tunnel to 125th St. Something about the shaking vibration of the train was unsettling, and the man, the man with the big voice behind me was making it worse.

OH NO NO NO NO NO!

My hip began to cramp up, and I began to shake lightly. I can't have this girl next to me see this! And her Mom will freak!

BUSINESS DUDE SHUT THE FUCK UP CAN'T YOU SEE I AM REGRESSING! I AM A CHILD AGAIN DON'T FUCKING HIT ME PLEASE!

I started to breathe quietly. I shut my eyes. I will breathe and I will sit here in my self-imposed darkness until it is safe to come out.

I felt trapped. I breathed. I prayed. I didn't move, but my body started to shake. I am not sure if the little girl or her mother saw me for I stayed in the darkness, eyes tight closed, hoping all would go away.

Forty five minutes later, we were almost at my stop, Goldens Bridge, where I would find my sanctuary, where it was safe to bounce and cry and howl with the demons from my past. But I had to get up, and Mommy and daughter were still there next to me. They must be going to Purdys or Carmel or somewhere far. Damn! I would have to get up. And when I get up I will start to bounce or fall over and I will scare this little girl next to me and most definitely her mother too. And maybe everyone on this train!

I think fast. I will write a letter. I pull out my bag. I am shaking. I pull out a spiral notebook and write a note:

I AM HAVING A PROBLEM WITH MY HIP AND I AM HAVING A HARD TIME WALKING AND I WILL BE SHAKING WHEN I GET UP AT MY STOP - GOLDENS

BRIDGE. I AM WRITING THIS NOTE TO YOU SO THAT I DON'T SCARE YOUR CHILD OR YOU. I AM FINE.

I sit for a moment. Should I give it to her? It is weird. But what is the alternative? Very weird. I give Mommy the note.

She reads it, looks furtively at me, and then nods. I smile. My head is shaking slightly side to side.

We arrive at Goldens Bridge. I nod to Mommy. She gets up with baby girl. I try to get up, great pain in my hip, and my body starts to shake. She looks at me in fear and turns her baby girl away. It seems like the whole train is looking at me as I shake like a cripple and make my way down the aisle, using the seats like crutches. Tears are streaming from my eyes. *I am a God Damn Leper! Oh please God why can't I just get off a train like a normal person?*

I exit the train. I lean against a poster for some bad Broadway play. The train pulls out. I wait. I wait until everyone leaves, and then I start my walk home.

I walk. I shake. My hip hurts. No one is watching. All is fine.

I get home.

I fall to the floor and pull my knees into my chest...

... and cry and cry and cry.

CHAPTER THIRTY-FIVE

I was a mess. My hip energy was moving side to side, from one hip to another, and I had this weird burning sensation in my back. I was in Marmaroneck, NY. I had just somehow made it through my morning workout classes pretending that I was OK. I talked through most of the class without demonstrating and I smiled a lot, but I was worried that at any moment my hip would lock up and I would start to shake, and my universe would explode. I stayed in HIGH ENERGY mode and I made it through the class.

As I was cleaning up, I knew I had to do something, and I also knew, I had to EAT. Eating was this bizarre way that I would manage my condition. Often by pigging out on really bad unhealthy yet delicious food, somehow that child part of me, Baby Ken, and the weird scary energy I called THE DARK MAN would simmer down. Usually it was sugar, usually in the form of cookies, cake or pie, but this particular day, it was PIZZA. My wacked out "inner child" who was now my "outer child" named Baby Ken and his dark nemesis, THE DARK MAN wanted PIZZA! And not just any Pizza, they wanted Sal's Pizza!

Sal's Pizza is legendary. His Sicilian pizza is baked twice, first with the amazing sauce, and then with the abundant cheese. The result is this utterly awesome, crisp, saucy, cheesy slice of Heaven. I needed some Heaven.

So that is how I ended up in Marmaroneck, NY, home to the amazing Sal's Pizza. I had three (count 'em), three slices.

After my smorgasbord of Italian delight, I went for a walk down the avenue. I was still a bit unsettled and walking often helped.

At the end of the avenue, there was a storefront with a small simple sign that read: "David Yu, Acupuncture - No appointment necessary." I stood for a moment in front of the store, and then a little voice inside me said:

"Go for it. What have you got to lose?"

I suddenly remembered when Alexander Hand did his crazy MOOBEE points on me and my world turned upside down. What if this acupuncture freed Baby Ken and The Dark Man? What if the NEEDLES manifested even more of this crazy energy in me?

I walked away.

I can't have that happen. No, I can't.

I walked to the top of the hill by a parking garage, and I turned around.

"Go for it."

It was that little voice.

"Go for it, Ken. The answer may lie with Mr. Yu."

I walked back and entered his storefront office. It was a large room that used to be a Jewelry store. Makeshift six foot tall cubicles lined up against one wall, all painted gray. There was a desk up front and a small office room in the back. Dirty gray carpeting. No one was there.

I waited.

Five minutes later, Dr. Yu appeared. I don't think he really was a Doctor but calling him a doctor in my head just felt better at the time.

He was small, about 5' 4" with jet black hair and a chiseled face.

"How may yai hep u?"

Oh no, this dude doesn't speak English. Hell, maybe there are Asian prostitutes in the back. This was not a good sign.

"Um I am uh having problems in my hips. It hurts… and it's tight." There was no way he would be able to understand my real story, and also no way he would ever understand my telling of it, so I kept it simple.

"I am tight here." And I pointed to my hip flexors.

"Ok Ok, I know. Yes, Ok go in hea please."

He pointed to one of the cubicles.

"Thanks."

"No ploblem. NO Ploblem."

"Oh yes PLOBLEM" I thought as I entered, "Oh Yes PLOBLEM!"

"Now take off shirlt and pant. Then Yai down pleas."

He pointed to a pink massage table. I slowly removed my shirt and pants, and lay down on the table.

"Ok now I put needle in. No ploblem, easy."

Time to go back to Sal's. I needed PIzza, or Gelato, or anything other than NEEDLES.

He took ten needles and put one in each of my ten toes. Then he placed three needles in each of my quads, four needles along my outer rib cage, and then finally at least eight needles in my crown of my head.

PLEASE PLEASE CHEESY HEAVEN SAL'S PLEASE!

Then he took a lone needle and stuck it into my solar plexus. With that prick, I immediately started to cry, and hyperventilate.

Oh no no please not now not again no not again!

"You Ok?" and then without even waiting for my response, he then attached an electrode to the pins connected to each of my pinky toes.

He is going to kill me!

"Now I turn on. Easy for you." He smiled.

I am going to woof my Sal's. I know it.

Dr. Yu turned on the juice. A light tingling sensation vibrated up my leg and then up my spine to the crown of my head.

"You Ok, good. I go away. Come back in half hour." And he left, just like that.

HALF HOUR? Thirty whole minutes? No No NO NO NO! I feel like Frankenstein on Heroin. Thirty minutes! Oh no please no!

My body continued to vibrate. I started to count backwards from 100 to 1. My toes were on fire. I could feel energy flowing up and down my body, and the tears fell, disconnected, but still vaguely painful like a long forgotten nightmare.

89, 88, 87, 86.

I squeezed all the muscles in my face for my head started to vibrate side to side, and I was fearful that I would jam a pin through my brain if I vibrated hard enough.

76, 75, 74, My left leg started to jump a bit.

Oh hell, my leg is going to jump and disconnect the juice.

57, 56, 55,

There was a warm feeling in my brain. Something was happening. How could I have a warm feeling in brain? A brain doesn't feel.

43, 42, 41, 40, 39

Please get me out of here, please get me out.
This is a Ploblem, a big Ploblem!

So I lay, and counted, and shuttered, and vibrated.

Please God let this work!

Twenty minutes later, Dr. Yu appeared. He shut off the juice and removed the pins.

"How you feel?"

I stopped for a moment to take notice of what was going on in my body. The energy in my body was moving. My hips seemed somehow clearer, not crystal clear, but clearer.

"I feel OK."

"Good, vely good, Ok is good. Tank you!"

"Tank you too."

I slowly get up off the massage table. I felt better, not perfect, but better.

It was time for PIE!

I walked down the block to Mozart's cafe, sat at a corner table. ordered a cafe mocha, and a huge slice of Apple Crumb pie.

Now I swear I didn't make this up. As I was consoling on the Apple Crumb pie, a little voice deep inside suddenly whispered to me.

THE ANSWER LIES IN YU! THE ANSWER LIES IN YU!

As I chomped down on my last forkful of Apple Crumb pie, I realized that there was something important here, maybe even the solution to The People in my Hips.

CHAPTER
THIRTY-SIX

My hips were feeling better, but they weren't better. There was some sort of odd energy release from what Dr. Yu did, but the energy was still there. The day after my first session with Dr. Yu, I felt great. But, by the end of the week, I was back to being locked up in my hips, with Baby Ken often causing me to shake. Luckily, the Dark Man didn't manifest. (*Oh please no!*) When the Dark Man came out to play, it was bad. It was like being stabbed by a harpoon in my right hip flexor.

So the following Monday, I decided to return to Dr. Yu to see if you could undo the energy again. It was the same deal. Ten pins in my toes, three pins in my quads, one pin in my solar plexus and 8 pins on my head. Again, my body started to vibrate, tears flew, and I lay there for thity minutes, while Dr. Yu wielded his energy magic with other devotees in the other cubicles. Thirty minutes later, he reappeared, unpinned me, and promptly said,

"Vely good. How you feel?"

"I feel good, I mean weird, but I feel better I think not all better but I think maybe I am a little maybe better."

He looked confused.

"What you say?"

"I feel better, yes I feel better."

"Vely Good. Energy maybe go away."

"I hope so. Why does this happen?"

He paused, squinted his eyes and said:

"I not see this offen but I see with Qi Gong. Many have too too too much enelgy - locked inside."

Qi Gong is a Chinese Yoga like practice which was banned by the Chinese government.

"Really, you have seen this?"

"Yes, many times, not here, in China I see what you have. Many times. Many times. Come you here please you?

He motioned for me to follow him to his office.

On the wall in his office was a big chart of the energy meridians in the body. He pointed to one of the lines.

"This is Liver melidian. Yours is blocked. Lots of enelgy stuck. You need to release. Acupuncture help."

I looked at the chart. The liver meridian comes up from the toes, up through the inner thigh and hip flexor, up into the lower back and liver and then up to the middle of the ribs by the solar plexus and then up the front of the neck, to the eyes and then the forehead.

It was almost exactly the areas where I was experiencing my crazy cramping and crazy energy flow.

WHAM! It was like an anvil was dropped on my head.

The answer lay not in stretching the areas where I was cramped up, like I had been doing for years with Yoga. The solution was in releasing the blocked areas <u>around</u> where I was cramping up, so the energy could flow!

BAM! WHAM! OUCH! THAT ANVIL HURTS!

No wonder the energy would flow left and right, left and right cramping my lower back and hip flexors. It was trapped between my rib cage and my quads.

My answer lie not in my PROBLEM - the cramped muscles, but in the ENVIRONMENT around it - the energy blocks at my ribcage and quads. If I could release those areas, possibly my symptoms would dissipate.
It was worth a try.

But the big question was this?

If this is just an energy block, why are BABY KEN and the DARK MAN living in my hips?

The whole paradigm of ENERGY release versus MUSCLE release was fascinating. I had been stretching the area where I was experiencing discomfort thinking that the discomfort was a cause of the tightness of the muscles, and at one level it was. But in reality, it was caused by the trapped energy in that area, causing my hip flexors and lower back to cramp. In actuality, to stretch the problem area actually released more energy, call it Trauma energy or Kundalini or Chi or whatever. So for three years, in my process to heal myself, I was actually releasing more energy in the problem area stretching those muscles, causing that area to continue to cramp. I was trapped in the conventional belief about what one should do with tight muscles - STRETCH!

DOES THIS MAKE ANY SENSE? You said it Sister!

So the key to my problem physically, was to release the BLOCKAGES that were preventing the energy to flow through my chakras or meridians or... well, hell, my body. If I could release those blockages, those areas outside of the problem area, possible, just possibly, I could release the energy and be healed.

The acupuncture had been effective to a point, but it never cleared my energy more than about 80%. I needed to somehow do more.

The idea hit me at the gym a couple days later. I was cramped up and I was hanging upside down on the stretch machine trying not to stretch my hip flexors too much when from that vantage point I saw one of those foam rollers that they have at gyms, often by the mat area. The rollers are made to release the fascia (the outer casing of muscles) in various parts of your body by literally rolling on this styrofoam thing. It was like a self massage. The question I asked myself from my bat-like upside-down position on the stretch machine was this:

WHAT IF I ROLLED OUT ON THE LIVER MERIDIAN?

Could it release more than the acupuncture?
Could it help clear this nasty energy out?

It was worth a try.

I jumped down, grabbed a long foam roller and made my way to a mat in the corner of the gym. It was mid afternoon so not so many people were around.
Thank God. I was not up to making a bouncing spectacle of myself.
I started by rolling the roller on my quads and immediately my head started to shake side to side.
Oh damn.
I then rolled over and started to roll on my upper lower back right where the muscles connect with my rib cage. My legs kicked up.
This is wild. This could be it. Damn. Keep going, Ken, keep going.

I rolled side to side on my lower back and my legs jumped and I started to cry, old painful trauma stuff but also DISCOVERY stuff, maybe this, god damnit, maybe this could finally be a solution. It was this weird mix of bad old pain and unbelievable hopeful joy. My body shook while I cried.

I then turned over and rolled on my solar plexus. My entire body bounced, shook, I cried and then I started to laugh, *yes maybe please please oh god thank you! - is this it? - please god please!*

I rolled for about 15 minutes.

The energy was definitely moving.

I took a shower and drove home, feeling like a million bucks. Like the old me, before all this happened.

That night, online, I ordered a foam roller of my own.

CHAPTER THIRTY-SEVEN

The Roller was like a drug, a good drug, a healthy drug, but an addictive drug just the same.

I became obsessed with rolling out my Chakras/ Meridians. As I rolled, I shook and bounced, vibrated and cried a bit, but every time within thirty minutes after rolling out, any pain or congestion or cramping would totally disappear. It was a miracle. A silly piece of styrofoam was my savior. Because of it, I was me again. No more fear that someone behind me would yell causing me to cramp up unexpectedly. No more fear of losing my job and my income because I was made a cripple from the Peeps. No more fear about my life. *NO MORE FEAR!*

And what was really cool too, was when the cramping and congestion disappeared so too would Baby Ken and The Dark Man, as if somehow they WERE that CRAMPING ENERGY, like the Black Smoke Monster from the TV show LOST.

All of a sudden, there was this opening in my life. There was clearly possibility again, possibility to be normal again, to be just like everyone else, no longer a Bouncing Leper with his heart on his hips.

So I lived with my Roller. That Summer, I actually took it and tennis balls on a trip to Bar Harbor, Maine. (I would roll on the tennis balls to release the energy.) Each morning and each night as I vacationed, I would roll out, to insure that nothing or no one, no SMOKE MONSTER would ruin my trip or my life.

It was a miracle.

That September, I stopped my therapy with Dr. Freud, and my one on one sessions with Douglass. That is when I also signed the lease on my new theatre, Manhattan Repertory Theatre, on 42nd St. in Manhattan. Life was so so so filled with possibility now. My old girlfriend Jen and I had recently hooked up again, and at last, THE WORLD WAS MY OYSTER, and boy, was I ready to eat.

I had fifteen blissful months of rolling out the Peeps, as I was producing and performing in new plays in our new theatre at night while working out and doing Yoga in classes and with private clients during the day. When my hips or my body got tight, I would roll out, shake a bit, and then all would be normal. It was working! Thank God, it was working!

Thank you, God. I am normal again.

And then, one week in late December, after rolling out my quads, lower back at the ribs and my solar plexus, the ENERGY, The BLACK SMOKE MONSTER, BABY KEN AND THE DARK MAN, wouldn't go away.

It stopped working. I have no idea why, but it stopped working. The energy actually got stronger and started to take over over my ENTIRE SPINE. I rolled out and out and out and out and out and ...NOTHING. It just got stronger. I was like a live wire channeling in EVERYTHING from my past, a million memories and feelings at once, and I knew it was old, but I could feel it and feel it and it wouldn't go away - the energy was so strong and ever present and *OH GOD NO NO NO PLEASE NO! !!!!!*

I WANT TO BE NORMAL! PLEASE!

It was coming out of every pore, following me, almost torturing me. I was undone, trying so desperately to hold on. Why was this memory, this energy, this person or persons, why were they in me and how the hell could I get them out?

YOU CAN'T COME BACK. I'M HAPPY! I AM BACK WITH JEN. ALL IS GOOD! I AM NORMAL! PLEASE, NO DON'T COME BACK! PLEASE NO!!!!

AHHHHHHHHHHHHHHHHHHHHHHHHHHHHH!!!!!

I tried rolling again and again, nothing.

I walked, ran around trying to dissipate the energy in my body...and nothing.

It was Christmas eve again.

And the Dark Man and Baby Ken were back...

...and it was party time!

CHAPTER THIRTY-EIGHT

They were there living in me, and on that day Christmas Eve, 2006, they had taken control of me. I had to do something. What what the hell could I do? Please God, help me!

And then I knew.

I would go home. Back to Yorktown. Where I grew up. And search for him. The Dark Man. That man who did something to me, something so horrendous that I pushed it into my body and out of my mind. I would go back to my home, and then let the People in my Hips find him! Yes, I know it was crazy, but what else could I do? I had to get this energy out of my body, Baby Ken and the Dark Man. It was time. Time to be free. Time to get them out once and for all and if it meant REMEMBERING THE DARK STUFF, I would do that.

I pulled my car out of the parking garage on 44th St. and headed toward the West Side Highway.

I had my lifeline with me. My little panasonic Video camera. I would film my journey. I would film my discoveries. I would make this happen.

My legs were shaking as I drove, and my head would shake occasionally all by itself. I was really scared. Some of it was old stuff, and some of it was present day fear, fear of what I might discover going back there, to the scene of the crime forty years earlier. I turned on the camera and talked as I drove.

"I am on the West Side Highway going up to Yorktown…" *Oh God please help me.*

It was a beautiful sunny winter day, cold and crisp. My little Green Honda Civic puttered along as I made my way up the West Side Highway to The Saw Mill Parkway to the Taconic State. At the Taconic State Parkway, I started to shake and my teeth started to chatter a bit. What the fuck was I doing? *NO NO NO NO NO NO! I had to get this HELL out of me. BABY KEN and the DARK MAN - I had to get them out. I wanted my life back, oh please please please.*

I turned on the carmera and talked. Talking to the camera grounded me. Kept me centered. Kept me focused. Who knows maybe some day this video will be on Oprah when I share this tale to the world. Maybe today, maybe today I will know and by knowing maybe I will be healed.

The search was on.

What if he was there, still alive after forty years.
He would have to be very old, but what if he were alive,
and I found him. What would I do? What could I do?
And what if he wanted to hurt me again?

I got images of pine trees and of a back porch and of
moldy wet smells. Damp. Cold. Could it be that house
across the street on Mark Rd? I would know soon enough.

I drove down the road that led to the development in
Yorktown where I lived. I was scared. Baby Ken was with
me and my right hip was throbbing. I am not ready to
listen to my hips, but I have to. I have to. It is time to be
free again.

I got to Edcris Rd. The road that I grew up on.
The road where I lived. The place where lots of things
happened, dark bad things, and even more I can't
remember, dark things that I stored in my hips.

It was time for my hips to talk.

I was surprisingly lucid now driving down the block.
I was curious, more curious than scared now. I drove
down the street. Gary Sabia's house, The Luperellos
House, Pagano's and then my house, our house, where I
grew up and made movies and put on puppet shows.
Where I smoked pot at thirteen and threw eggs off the
roof on Halloween at the passing cars. The house, my

home where I grew up, where I learned to be creative to deal with the madness around me.

As I drove by, I felt nothing in my hips. It was quiet. I drove down Mark Rd past the house where something may have happened. Nothing. Nothing. *What? NO please no! I need this out of me. Out of me!*

I turned the car around. I was talking to the video camera now. I am feeling nothing and then…

My body started to bounce, *oh my God it was here, something happened here, Baby Ken was with me now and he was scared, we were both together, both of us!*

I pulled over.

What happened here? What happened? Talk to me! Talk to me.

We are both in my consciousness - Baby Ken is scared so so scared.

Talk to me. Talk to me. What happened?

My face is twisted. We are both here. The Dark Man in my right hip is there too.

What happpened? Talk to me! Talk to me. What happened?

He is right with me. Baby Ken. We are one. What happened?

My God, it was forty years ago!

IT WAS FORTY YEARS AGO!
IT WAS FORTY YEARS AGO!

It was forty years ago.

Baby Ken heard me.
He was here now in 2006, not 1966.
There was no Dark Man here.
No one.

Just a video camera and a green Honda Civic driving
through an old development.

There was no Dark Man here.
It was 2006.
Christmas Eve.
The Dark Man was gone.
Probably died.
I/Baby Ken don't belong here.
I have grown up.....
I wept.

Something happened just then.
I didn't know what.

But Baby Ken, the Dark Man, the shaking, the fear.. was somehow transformed into the tears of a forty-eight year old man...

      ...quietly sobbing alone in his car.

CHAPTER THIRTY-NINE

In that moment, on Christmas eve 2006, in that peak emotional moment, Baby Ken and I connected. Baby Ken finally understood that it happened forty years ago.
The present suddenly became safe, and Baby Ken and The Dark Man were sent back in time, where they belong:

The PAST. Yesterday. Forty years ago.

Since that fateful day, I have had no communication with Baby Ken or the Dark Man and virtually no Post Traumatic Stress Disorder Symptoms.

In that moment, while desperately following my intuition and my hips in Yorktown Heights, I was cured.

I didn't remember what happened. And I was cured. In conventional therapy, it is in the "remembering" that often people are cured. But I didn't remember. I didn't remember anything about "the event" and I was cured.

And I didn't care. The Peeps were gone.

Damn, I was happy!

Since my cure, I went on to create my one man show THE PEOPLE IN MY HIPS which outlined this tale, with acted out scenes, candid narration and with real video from this experience, which was performed for four months in 2009 at my theatre, Manhattan Repertory Theatre in New York City. It was scary sharing this experience, but worth it for I received rave reviews. I then went on to blog the entire PEEPS story with more video in greater detail at: www.thepeopleinmyhips.com.

And then, one day in September 2010, while sitting with my MacBook Pro at Starbucks in Rye, New York, I ran into my younger sister Margie. I was talking about The People in my Hips blog and about possibly doing The People in my Hips play again when she said to me:

"I think I know who the Dark Man is."

"What?" I replied semi-stunned.

"I think I know who the Dark Man is."

"How?"

"I have been doing some therapy. EMDR. Working on my relationship issues. And I remembered something. I think I know who he is."

"Tell me, please. Tell me."

"No, I can't right now. I have to go to work but let's find time to talk and I will tell you the story."

So that Saturday, we met at the Starbucks in Rye, NY and walked down to the park by the library. Sitting on a green park bench together, Margie shared her amazing tale.

But how could Margie know? It was forty years ago when the DARK MAN perpetrated his madness on me and forty years ago when I locked that traumatic memory deep in my subconscious mind and in the muscles of my body. How could Margie know? I didn't even know and I was there. I had sifted through the sand of my unconscious for years. All I had were brief frightening images, (trees, a porch, a balding man with squinty eyes, walking home and being so scared to tell anyone for fear I would be murdered) and the crazy somatic responses in my body while I was involved in my People in Hips journey (hands on my neck, being hit repeatedly on my back and all over my body, and an automatic bouncing of my body that seemed as if I was being raped.)

Now Margie, my dear and wonderful sister, was going to tell me what happened forty years ago.

I am crying as I write this for this is the conclusion. I thought putting it away in a box in my past was enough, and it is enough to prevent the PTSD, to prevent the shaking, to prevent the spontaneous cramping of my hip flexors and to keep Baby Ken and the Dark Man in my unconscious at bay. It's enough. Putting it in a box in the past works. It relieves the pain, the present day pain. There is no baby Ken here, no Dark Man. They are and were manifestations of my past, my trauma, my lost childhood.

But now, knowing the truth seems somehow… sublime.

It is said that the truth will set you free, and in my case, it will. It will set me free from the fear of not knowing, free from the fear of being crazy and free from the fear of Baby Ken and The Dark Man returning someday for even more fun. The truth will firmly seat me in my body, validating my People in my Hips experience as being real.

After all this, I like real.

Now Margie was going to tell me what happened.

Forty years ago.

Amazing.

CHAPTER
FORTY

"I have been in therapy trying to figure out why for most of my life I have been in relationships with men who needed my help. Men who had mental problems, men who couldn't keep it together, men who weren't there for me and couldn't be because of problems that they had. And most importantly, we were trying to figure out why I felt compelled to help them. We were doing EMDR therapy with my therapist where I am put into sort of a hypnotic trance and we go back to get to the root of my issues and this is what I remembered: I was maybe eight years old, and I am walking up Mark Road in Yorktown, right by our house, and I hear yelling, arguing coming from down the hill by the house across the street. (The same house that my hip lead me to on December 24, 2006 - the day I was cured of my PEEPS condition.) I walked further up the road where I could see what was happening down behind the house."

Margie was visibly upset, on the verge of tears.

"You were there." she continued, "You were yelling, wearing a red plaid shirt, your hair parted at the side. And a MAN was yelling back at you. Balding. Dark squinty eyes. Partially graying. He was standing on his back porch. It was Mr. Kirkpatrick."

My mind reeled. I don't remember <u>and</u> it makes sense.

Yes. That porch. That porch, the one I remembered so often in Yoga, that porch connected with so so so so much fear. She continues with her story. I see it in my mind's eye.

"I can walk through your yard anytime I want." I said defiantly.

"Oh no you can't." The Dark Man yelled back.

"I am just taking the path down through the woods." (Yes, those woods the woods that I remembered so often in fear.)

"Get out of there! Get off my property!

"I will do what I want." Egging him on like I egged on my father. "What are you going to do about it?

There was an aluminum bat, with a red handle and a silver top. It was in his hand. He came at me.

"LEAVE ME ALONE, GOD DAMNIT! GET AWAY!"

And then, she saw this man, this DARK MAN, this god damned fucking monster of humanity come at me. As I turn to run, he hits me in the back of my left knee with the bat. I fall against a big pine tree, and THE DARK MAN starts to beat me repeatedly as I scream in terror.

THE DARK MAN stops a moment and turns, and sees Margie watching in terror, so Margie runs and runs and runs, terror racing through her veins. She runs and runs and runs to get help but she is so scared - she doesn't know what to do, she is so so so so crazy scared she needs to help me but she can't!

Should I go to a neighbors house? please god oh please someone help me help my brother down the hill he is going to die but I don't know what to do Oh please please help!

A woman runs out from the house and grabs her. It is our neighbor's wife.

"If you tell anyone, you will get hurt."

My sister pulls away. Her shoe gets caught by the street curb and falls off and she runs away in terror up to our house, up to safety. As she gets to our driveway, she sees him. Our EVIL NEIGHBOR - THE DARK MAN. He is like an animal, angry, crazy angry nuts angry out of his mind. An animal hunting his prey. With dark squinty evil eyes. He grabs her. Throws her down.

"DON'T YOU TELL ANYONE!"

He tears some grass from the lawn and shoves it in her mouth. And then, he stops. He hears something. Is it a neighbor? He runs away. Away to safety and the bad boy who dared to walk through his lawn who will pay for his transgression.

HE WILL PAY FOR WALKING THROUGH MY YARD!

Margie is standing now in the park in Rye, tears streaming down her face, her body shaking. She is back there, reliving it as she continues her tale.

"So I ran. I am so sorry. I ran away. I thought they were going to come and get me. I ran and ran and ran. I didn't know what to do. I didn't know what to do. So I ran around the block, through yards, down to the cul de sac on Sherry St. I found some bushes and I hid in the bushes. And I was so scared for you. I wanted to help you but I had to hide. I was scared. Finally, maybe thirty forty minutes later, I walked back. I had to see if you were ok. I left you. I had to see if you were OK."

Margie stood there weeping, by our green park bench, like a lost little girl.

"So I walk back. I was so scared.... And then I saw you, walking up to our house. You were hurt. And I couldn't help. I watched you go up to the house. You were hurt."

In that moment, an image, a strange image came back that had manifested in that therapy session, so many years before, when I realized that THE DARK MAN was trapped with Baby Ken in my body. It was the image of walking up to our house, knowing I had to keep it a secret or I would be killed.

What better way to keep a secret:
MAKE YOURSELF FORGET.

It matched her story.

She was there.

It was real.

CHAPTER FORTY-ONE

Margie was weeping now. Trembling.

"Ken, I'm so sorry. I'm so sorry. Can you ever forgive me? Can you please forgive me? I am so sorry. Please please forgive me!"

"Yes, Marge, of course I forgive you. It was forty years ago, I am fine."

"Please please please forgive me. I am so sorry."

"You didn't do anything wrong. He did. He was evil. He was wrong. You did your best. Your very very best. I love you."

I hugged her softly, and she wept in my arms.

This event, which we both pushed deep into our unconscious minds, (and in my case, my body) changed the course of our lives.

Margie spent the rest of her life, up until that moment in that park in Rye, NY, unconsciously compelled to help or save EVERYONE in her life for she was unable to help me on that oh so dark day, forty years ago.

Oh God Margie, I am so sorry.

And I, by the DARK MAN, was given the curse of
The People in my Hips.

One event changed the course of our lives. I thought
this was my story, but the miracle and tragedy here is, it
wasn't. This tale, my tale... is shared. Someone was there.
My amazing sister Margie was there.

Oh God, it was real.

I vaguely remember the incident behind the Dark
Man's house. The somatic feelings of getting hit on my
back when the People in my Hips first manifested big
time, now made sense. I was beat on my back by an
aluminum bat. The somatic hands on my throat must have
been his, and the memory of being held down when I
had the Moobee points done on me by Alexander Hand,
must have also been from this experience.

And then there was the somatic memory of being
raped which showed up in Yoga. Did that happen that
day when my sister ran away?

I don't know. I can't remember.

...and it's better that way.

The next day, I received a phone call from my sister She found out information about The Dark Man and she found a picture from 1963, all by searching the internet. In the picture she found, he was balding with dark squinty eyes.

It was him.

But now, The Dark Man was dead.

He died just about four years ago, in 2007, in a car accident.

He can't hurt me, or my sister, ever again.

But on that day, that fateful day, Christmas Eve 2006, when I followed my hip to Yorktown and was miraculously cured...

        ...I was parked in front of his house.

And at the time, he was alive. He was probably sitting in his house, less than 30 yards away.

The world works in mysterious ways.

CHAPTER
FORTY-TWO

It's been a little over four years since my final meeting with Baby Ken and the Dark Man, and my spontaneous and desperate journey back to Yorktown.

I'm better than ever. Emotionally and otherwise.

And every morning, when I wake up, and look over at my beautiful girlfriend, Jennifer, and our gorgeous puppy, Roma, I thank God that I am waking up "alone."

There is a sense of peace in me now, a sense of calm in knowing that no matter what happens to me in this life, there is a still strong voice inside me, call it my soul, call it my true self, or call it God, but no matter what you call it, this voice will always be there to guide me, take care of me, and carry me through any and all adversity.

Will I ever get on Oprah with this tale? I don't know and I really don't care. My mission now is to get the word out about the possibilities surrounding mental disease and Post Traumatic Stress Disorder and if Oprah wants to help, I would be thrilled, but I can't wait for her to get on

The People in my Hips bandwagon. It is time to get the word out, and there is no time like THE PRESENT.

When I first performed my one man show The People in my Hips, at the end of the play, I had a gift for every member of the audience. It was the official:

PEOPLE IN MY HIPS

(I - ain't - ever - going - there!)

ASHTRAY!

Soon, I will be selling them online.

There are circles within circles in this life we live.

Sometimes the circles complete quickly, and sometimes the circles take forty years, but I have this firm belief that before we embrace our maker,

EVERYTHING is resolved.

And then, we move on.

My People in my Hips journey is far from over. It is time for me to get this story out to the world at large to challenge today's rather archaic models of mental health and solutions for Post Traumatic Stress Disorder.

The mind and the body are infinitely connected, and mental health strategies need to be re-thought with this in mind, so that more of those afflicted can recover fully and live happier, healthier lives.

My journey to the edge of what our society calls "madness" forced me to grow, change, and now, to live more fully in the present moment, and for that opportunity, I thank The People in my Hips, and more importantly, I thank that still strong voice inside me, that guided me back to health, balance, and ultimately, back into the light.

AFTERWARD

If you know anyone who experiences symptoms of PTSD, random anxiety, depression or other symptoms of powerful emotions manifesting out of what seems like nothing, please have them contact me at:

thepeopleinmyhips@gmail.com

I might be able to help.

Also you can check out my blog, (from which this book was based) at: www.thepeopleinmyhips.com

There, you will find this story in a slightly different form, and you will also find scores of entries about Yoga, emotion and energy with lots of real video of my People in my Hips adventure.

In any given moment in time,
            there is possibility for change.

Wishing you light, love and prosperity!

Ken Wolf
March 5, 2011
New York City

Special Thanks

Without the profound help and support of Yogi
Douglass Stewart, and psychologist Dr. Brian Healy,
I wouldn't be here today. I cannot even begin to express
how thankful I am for their support and gentle guidance
during my People in my Hips adventure.

Also, profound, everlasting love and great thanks to
the love of my life, Jennifer Pierro, who stuck with me
through the process, even as our world imploded.
Thanks to my brother Mike for always being there,
and extra special thanks to my incredible and amazing
sister Margie, who helped me put together the last piece
of my People in my Hips puzzle. I love you all dearly.

Lastly, I would like to thank God for leading me down
this crazy path to wholeness.

I am no longer run by my past.

I am here, living fully in the present,

...and so damn happy just to be alive.

www.ingramcontent.com/pod-product-compliance
Lightning Source LLC
Chambersburg PA
CBHW061403280526
45784CB00001B/358